HOW TO PREVENT DIABETES

Motivate yourself not to become statistic

Dorris S. Woods, Phd

Library of Congress Control Number: 2023919559
            Paperback: 979-8-9886071-7-5

In Praise and Support of How to Prevent Diabetes- *I Beat It and You Can, Too!*

First she gave us the ground-breaking report on teenage suicides with her book *Breaking Point: Fighting to End America's Teenage Suicide Epidemic.*
Now author Dorris S. Woods, Ph.D. RN, CS has again enlightened us on the connection between obesity and diabetes with her latest book entitled *How to Prevent Diabetes - I Beat It and You Can, Too!*

Her conversational dialogue throughout the book easily leads you through her winning strategies for fighting the fastest growing health epidemic in our country. Her writing successfully holds your attention on the subject.

I would recommend this latest publication as a must-read text for lay persons, looking to do something about this national health crisis and for health professionals and students of the health field. The topic is high on the agenda even of our first lady, Michele Obama. Embrace this book to implement your own personal plan for avoiding this health problem and pass on a copy to a friend or relative as a positive step toward solving this poor health trend. I wholeheartedly endorse this read.

- Patricia Shade, Esq.

Dr. Woods and I concur that lifestyle changes are important in the treatment and prevention of diabetes. The changes need to have staying power, that is that one changes, and stays changed.

- Gloria Allen, BS, MS, Research Consultant, University of Southern California (USC)

A simple guide for losing weight and maintaining a healthier lifestyle.

- Mary J. Smith, Commentator

Book is clear and direct. Can be very helpful to any reader, who buys and reads it.

- Diane Raintree, Editor

How to Prevent Diabetes – I Beat It and You Can, Too!

DORRIS S. WOODS, PH.D., RN, CS

My determination not to become a statistic was an excellent decision.
Simple lifestyle changes have made all the difference.
Slender thighs, a flat belly, control of my "bat wings" and firm buttocks have made it more than worthwhile.
I'm happy with the world on a string.

- Dorris S. Woods, Author

To my husband and son,
Dr. Burton L. Woods
and
Dr. Brannon L. Woods
Who always encouraged me to lose the weight.
You're gone, but never forgotten.

Acknowledgments

A debt of gratitude is owed to everyone who impacted the writing of this book.

My profound gratitude goes to my endocrinologist, Dr. Susan Davis. Her proactive approach to disease prevention is appreciated.

Her approach provided the impetus for me to work toward becoming a healthier person, increasing my learning curve about food and exercise and hopefully preventing Diabetes Type II.

I am also grateful for the information and encouragement that Pamela Lee, RD provided in the initial stages. Had I followed what she said and had written it down the food chosen when eating out, would have made my weight loss efforts more successful. Instead, I procrastinated for too long.

My friend, Gloria Allen, has shared her family's genetic connection to diabetes. She is supportive for the writing of this book, along with everyone who is aware that it is being written. Many have requested copies for family members.

I am most grateful for Mr. Thomas Mulligan's patience with all the changes made as research and learning improved.

To my Grady colleagues, who were concerned that I need not write another "diet book," I say that the time and effort that went into being the guinea pig for the information in the book was well worth it, having saved me from myself. Hopefully, it will inspire others to try and prevent diabetes, and, most importantly encourage physicians to take a proactive approach, as Dr. Davis did, rather than the reactive approach to treat the disease after it is contracted.

Foreword

How to Prevent Diabetes - I Beat It and You Can, Too, tells the true story of the author's determination not to become a statistic in America's epidemic of Type II Diabetes.

Cultural changes in the United States have caused a pandemic level of obese individuals, the author being one of them. The obesity has triggered an epidemic of diabetes. While diabetes can be controlled once a diagnosis is made, the condition may cause serious health problems with the eyes, kidneys, nervous system, feet, skin, teeth and gums. The most serious problems for women are those that lead to amputations, heart disease, heart attacks, and strokes.

Although my story is true, it's not unique, because the "prediabetic" diagnosis was made by an alert doctor, not because I'd experienced symptoms. Many diabetics are identified during routine physical exams.

Once I learned of my problem, the challenge was to make changes to my current lifestyle in terms of nutrition and exercise. The choices I made may not be those that work for someone else, but do provide a blueprint for change.

My success is due to the concept of staying power. Staying power means long-term, positive changes needed to achieve a goal. In other words, exercising and losing weight are great for change with a sense of permanence intended. I needed to change and stay changed.

Staying power has given me "bragging rights." The A1C is a measure of the average blood glucose level over a three-month period. A reading above 6.0 is cause for action to prevent it from going higher. My A1C, the gold standard for diabetic testing, has remained at 5.3

for more than a year, even 5.2 at one point. Dr. Susan Davis, my endocrinologist at the University of California, Los Angeles (UCLA), told me, "You've set the standard. Now it's up to you to maintain it. It's probably as good as or better than anyone on staff." Pamela Lee, the dietitian, said that typically when a patient's A1C is initially given, it goes up rather than down. I work at making mine lower and keeping it there.

The purpose of this book is to share my story of success and to encourage the millions of people who don't know that they are diabetic to get tested.

Happy reading!

Table of Contents

Chapter 1

The Day I Got
Scared Straight

Diet and exercise. There are no shortcuts.

- Lisa Masterson, M.D.
"The Doctors" TV Show

AS THE CHRISTMAS HOLIDAY grew closer, I was excited about my trip to Chicago for a visit with my brother and his family. One particular day I really did not have time to keep my appointment with my endocrinologist, Dr. Susan Davis. However, as a professional registered nurse, I recognized the importance of the visit. Besides, she always has an unbelievably busy schedule and rescheduling was not a smart move.

My previous visits were aimed at regulating my thyroid medication. The blood work that provided Dr. Davis with the data she needed to make a determination had been done the previous week. What I had not considered was that she had much more data than just the blood work for the thyroid.

In addition to a thyroid problem, I had been overweight for the second half of my life, along with borderline hypertension. So, when I went in for this visit, I expected some reference to my weight problem or blood pressure. But when Dr. Davis said, "You know, you're borderline diabetic," my mouth fell open. I was speechless, in shock. I did not believe, or rather, did not want to believe, what I had just heard, as though I was invincible.

"See," she said, pointing to the lab slip and the analysis.

Yes, I saw it, written in black and white. However, the data did not register with me, because I did not want to hear about it. I felt disgusted with myself, and the fact that Dr. Davis told me was good enough. I do recall that my blood sugar and A1C were above-normal. I do not remember the numbers.

A mild depression set in, as I left her office with the firm determination that I would do something about turning around my situation. Dr. Davis had told me, in essence: "Lose some weight and exercise." It was that simple.

I left for Chicago shortly after my visit to Dr. Davis' office. During the flight my thoughts drifted back: many decades ago to when I was a student nurse at Grady Memorial Hospital in Atlanta. This large hospital for the indigent was located on the southeast side of the city near the Centers for Disease Control. We had many obese diabetics on every service. My thoughts were of "them" being diabetic, not me.

At the moment my priority was how to manage all the Christmas goodies and prevent a bigger problem for myself while on holiday. I resolved that the time was now, beginning with the treats on the flight.

However, I could still visualize patients having circulatory problems in their lower extremities. Gangrene sometimes sets in and amputations became necessary. Some came into the hospital because the diabetes was out of control. Insulin and diet needed to be regulated to prevent diabetic coma or acidosis. Acidosis occurs when body chemistry becomes imbalanced and overly acidic. Pregnant women were always at high risk for gestational diabetes. The patients who had surgery had wounds that were slow to heal.

Although I did not recall everything that occurred during my training, I specifically did not remember emphasizing exercise and weight control while advising patients.

I stayed in Chicago for a week and despite all the holiday treats and dishes we prepared, I lost two pounds and was very pleased. My willpower kicked in, and I limited my intake of pie, cake, cornbread and other sugar and starches. I made a mindful effort to eat meat and vegetables. I was also able to do some exercises in my room, and drank water.

Upon my return home I kept my appointment with the dietitian. We reviewed my overeating, lack of exercise, and major specific food weaknesses. When she brought out her teaching tools (e.g., measuring cups, spoons) I was again surprised by the amount of one cup. I just about flipped. "What?" I asked her. For a person who ordinarily ate a bed of rice amounting to at least 2-1/2 cups and filled her cereal bowl to the brim, this sudden awareness was a big deal. I had to give serious thought to the amount of food I was consuming.

We actually talked about the empty calories in white rice. She said, "Brown rice is a better choice," reminding me that the choice of foods also makes a difference.

Although I liked rice a lot, my big addiction was peanuts. I could buy Planter's peanuts by the jar and finish off half of it, while just driving home from the market. Peanuts were my favorite snack, with or without raisins.

My history with a peanut addiction extended over several decades. If I did not hide my stash from my husband, he would toss them out. After he passed on, my son Brannon took up the cause. Being a confirmed practical joker, he once gave me a gallon of peanuts at Christmas. After I saw the container, the peanuts disappeared without any explanation. I realized that both my husband and son were trying to help me. Peanuts are not necessarily a non-healthy snack, but I just ate too many at one time. They are both gone now, so it is up to me to get the job done. I will not disappoint them.

Getting back to my dietitian's visit and the issue with peanuts, she said that there was no good reason to entirely omit foods from the diet, just use moderation. For once I made a firm decision about peanuts: I would limit myself to peanuts in the shells to a half cup at my mid- afternoon snack. Surprisingly, I found this amount quite satisfying.

I was pleased with the advice given to me, because the amount of food was not measured by calorie counting. Measuring became easier.

After losing twelve pounds I was off "borderline diabetes II" in just one month. I continued the learning process and lost 40 pounds in six months. I had a non-age-related hip problem that led to a prescription for Prednisone, causing difficulty in losing weight and exercising. This particular prescription inevitably caused weight gain. However, not having the information about food management would have caused me to gain excess weight. I tend to empathize with problem weight watchers, as I have been one.

Today I have captured the essence of what you can do to lose weight and never again diet. During the process of learning how to lose the weight, you also learn how to maintain normal healthy weight. Your learning curve goes up and you are there. If you occasionally "fall off the wagon," do not go around beating up on yourself, but simply start back where you left off as soon as you can. You do not have to confine yourself to special foods; just learn to eat sensibly. After a while your bad habits change and good eating habits take hold with no diet, pills, injections, or surgery. Simply use a little willpower. The stomach will shrink in size and less food is desired.

Just as we plan for a successful job experience or career, we can also plan a successful weight-management lifestyle.

Making a Diabetic Diagnosis

One may have type 2 diabetes and not know it. Sometimes type 2 diabetes has no warning signs at all. Therefore, blood plasma glucose levels are important for identifying both diabetes and pre-diabetes.

Normal blood plasma glucose levels	70-99 mg/dl
Pre-diabetes blood plasma glucose levels	100-125 mg/dl
Diabetes blood plasma glucose levels	126 mg/dl or more on more than one test

The normal, pre-diabetic or diabetic diagnosis is confirmed by laboratory tests on the blood plasma glucose levels:

(1) A fasting specimen for glucose level is done after 8 hours of not eating or drinking.

(2) A glucose tolerance test measures your blood glucose level after you have gone 8 hours without eating and 2 hours after you drink a glucose-containing beverage.

(3) A random blood plasma glucose test to measure your blood glucose at any time of the day. The doctor will ask you about diabetic symptoms.

Source: *The Healthy Woman*
        U.S. Department of Health and Human Services, 2011, pp. 72-73

CHAPTER 2

Being "Fat" Is a
Diabetes Risk

Taking charge of your life is deeply satisfying.

- Rose Marie Robinson, M.D.

UPON RETURNING FROM CHICAGO, I was well aware that decisive action had to be taken for reducing my weight. I was surprised to learn that obesity is a major contributing factor in the rise of Diabetes Type II.

My body mass index (BMI) was over 40, as I weighed more than 240 pounds. The BMI is a calculation using weight and height to determine how much of your weight is from fat. The higher the BMI, the greater the excess fat, and thus, the greater the risk of developing diabetes, especially when other risk factors are present.

A person's weight is considered healthy if the BMI is 19-24.9; moderately healthy if the BMI is 25-29.9; and a BMI over 30 is classified as obese. The numbers are indicators of the amount of fat present in the body. I had known for some time that I was overweight, being 100 pounds above normal weight. I just neglected to do something about it and was aware of the genetic propensity toward diabetes.

People whose BMI's are at a healthy level do not experience organ failure at the same rate as those whose BMI is beyond 30 and who are diabetic.

The body loses its sensitivity to insulin in Diabetes II. Insulin is

What's Your BMI?

To learn BMI, just use the following chart.* First, find your height in the left column.

Then, read along the row for your height until you reach the weight closest to yours.

Finally, move straight up the chart to find your BMI.

Body Mass Index

Height	19	20	21	22	23	24	25	26	27	28	29	30	31	32	33	34	35	36	37	38	39	40
4'10"	91	95	100	105	110	114	119	124	129	133	139	143	148	152	157	162	167	172	176	181	186	191
4'11"	94	99	104	104	114	119	124	129	134	139	144	149	154	159	164	169	174	179	184	188	193	198
5'	97	102	107	112	117	122	127	132	138	143	148	153	158	163	168	173	178	183	188	194	199	204
5'1"	101	106	111	117	122	127	132	138	143	148	154	159	164	169	175	180	185	191	196	201	207	212
5'2"	103	109	114	120	125	130	136	141	147	152	158	163	168	174	179	185	190	196	201	206	212	217
5'3"	107	113	119	124	130	135	141	147	152	158	164	169	175	181	186	192	198	203	209	214	220	226
5'4"	111	117	123	129	135	141	146	152	158	164	170	176	182	187	193	199	205	211	217	223	228	234
5'5"	114	120	126	132	138	144	150	156	162	168	174	180	186	192	198	204	210	216	222	228	234	240
5'6"	118	124	131	137	143	149	156	162	168	174	180	187	193	199	205	212	218	224	230	236	243	249
5'7"	121	127	134	140	147	153	159	166	172	178	185	191	196	204	210	217	223	229	236	242	248	255
5'8"	125	132	139	146	152	158	165	172	178	185	191	198	205	211	218	224	231	238	244	251	257	264
5'9"	128	135	142	149	155	162	169	176	182	189	196	203	209	216	223	230	236	243	250	257	263	270
5'10"	133	140	147	154	161	168	175	182	189	196	203	210	217	224	231	237	244	251	258	265	272	279
5'11"	136	143	150	157	164	171	179	186	193	200	207	214	221	229	236	243	250	257	264	271	279	286
6'	140	148	155	162	170	177	185	192	199	207	214	221	229	236	244	251	258	266	273	281	288	295
6'1"	143	151	158	166	174	181	189	196	204	211	219	226	234	241	249	257	264	272	279	287	294	302
6'2"	148	156	164	171	179	187	195	203	210	218	226	234	242	249	257	265	273	281	288	296	304	312
6'3"	151	159	167	175	183	191	199	207	215	223	231	239	247	255	263	271	279	287	294	302	310	318
6'4"	156	164	172	181	189	197	205	214	222	230	238	246	255	263	271	279	287	296	304	312	320	328

*Adapted from "Clinical Guidelines on the Identification, Evaluation, and Treatment of Overweight and Obesity in Adults," NIH Publication No. 98-4083, September 1999. National Institutes of Health.

a hormone secreted by the pancreas that is responsible for helping muscles absorb and use blood sugar glucose. The insulin "unlocks" cell walls to let glucose into the cells, providing energy for the body. If the cells fail to respond properly to insulin, "resistance" causes some cells to not receive glucose for energy. If the insulin is unable to allow the glucose into the cells, it remains in the bloodstream or spills into the kidneys. Both these cases can lead to serious problems if untreated. Too much body fat interferes with insulin's ability to allow or "unlock" cells.

During my learning process I had almost every risk factor for developing diabetes. In addition to being obese, I am over 45 years of age; and not particularly active physically. My mother had diabetes and died of heart failure; my two brothers, one sister and a nephew have the condition; lastly, I am African American with high blood pressure. African-Americans have diabetes at a high rate and suffer from many of the effects of the disease such as strokes, heart failure, kidney failure, cataracts, blindness, peripheral neuropathy or nerve damage of the lower extremities and high blood pressure.

Whatever the role fat and other risk factors play, I cannot ignore the influence heredity plays in causing diabetes in African-Americans and especially in my own family (see chart). My mother was diabetic, bore me, a prediabetic, and my sister, June, who is a "brittle" diabetic, meaning she easily fluctuates from high to low blood sugar and is insulin-dependent. June must have nine lives like a cat. Several times already she has had a blood sugar too high to read, followed by a blood glucose of 22, 27, and 33. She can feel the symptoms coming on but is unable to control them. Sometimes she will fight like a mad person. Doctors are not able to determine the exact cause of her glucose-insulin problem, but it appears to be related to a lack of muscle tissue to properly transport insulin. June's son, Micky, was recently diagnosed with diabetes. Cataracts had developed in Micky to the point where the doctor wondered how he could see to drive. Micky had not had a physical for many, many years after a serious accident. His blood sugar was 361, 262 above normal. In addition to June and her son Micky being diabetic, my two brothers also have the disease.

Lynell has had diabetes for years. Then Gary was diagnosed within the past year, when he went to the doctor to have a "boil" on his leg treated. He mentioned to the doctor that he had "blurred" vision as well, like Micky. A lab test showed that he had a blood glucose of 475.

He was told that he was a "ticking time bomb." The doctor almost hospitalized him on the spot.

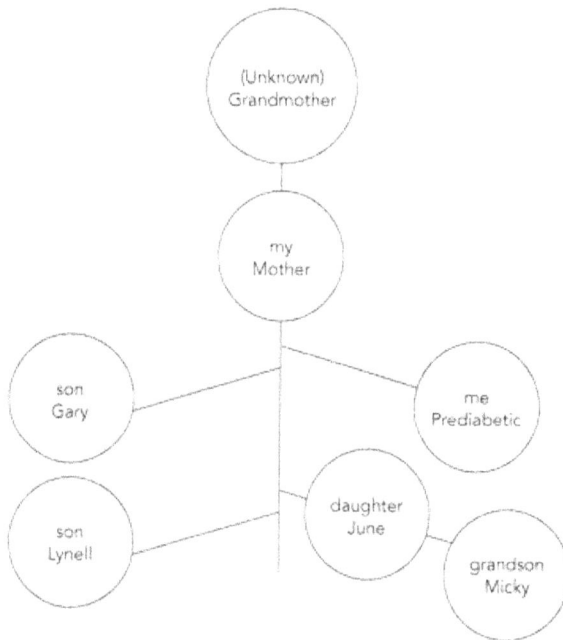

My grandmother died, when my mother was a young child. The cause of death was not known. I do know that her father died from natural causes. Most probably the diabetic gene was transmitted from the mother.

"Did you know Bernice had a stroke?" Gussie asked me recently.

"No," I replied. "When did it happen?"

"Since we came from the family reunion," she said. "But listen to this: Bernice is diabetic, but when she went for her diabetic teaching, she had the nurse teach Bernadette how to do the insulin injections. She said that she couldn't stick herself. Bernadette gets up early to go to work and leaves Bernice asleep. Bernice was not getting her insulin.

"When she was taken to the hospital she had a left-side stroke with paralysis. Her blood sugar was over 400. She is walking wobbly, but still can't give her own insulin, because she is left-handed and can't hold the syringe."

Gussie, the sister-in-law talking with me, is also diabetic, but controls it with pills, diet, and exercise. Gussie's left knee is a a problem. She has gained about 15 pounds, but is being as active as possible and watching what she eats.

Gussie's and Bernice's mother, my mother-in-law, died of diabetic complications. So diabetes certainly runs in the family. My brothers-in-law, Bill and Richard, are also diabetic, but are much disciplined and have few problems with the disease (see two diagrams).

In my biological family, also from Mississippi like my husband's, my mother was diabetic and died of a heart attack at 93. She was a

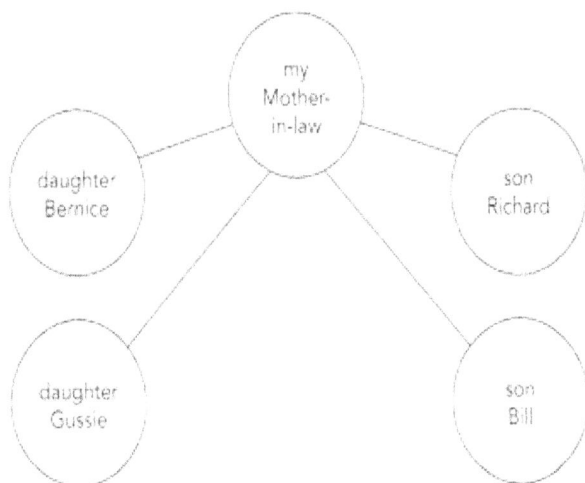

"Did you know Bernice had a stroke?" Gussie asked me recently.

"No," I replied. "When did it happen?"

"Since we came from the family reunion," she said. "But listen to this: Bernice is diabetic, but when she went for her diabetic teaching, she had the nurse teach Bernadette how to do the insulin injections. She said that she couldn't stick herself. Bernadette gets up early to go to work and leaves Bernice asleep. Bernice was not getting her insulin.

"When she was taken to the hospital she had a left-side stroke with paralysis. Her blood sugar was over 400. She is walking wobbly, but still can't give her own insulin, because she is left-handed and can't hold the syringe."

Gussie, the sister-in-law talking with me, is also diabetic, but controls it with pills, diet, and exercise. Gussie's left knee is a a problem. She has gained about 15 pounds, but is being as active as possible and watching what she eats.

Gussie's and Bernice's mother, my mother-in-law, died of diabetic complications. So diabetes certainly runs in the family. My brothers-in-law, Bill and Richard, are also diabetic, but are much disciplined and have few problems with the disease (see two diagrams).

In my biological family, also from Mississippi like my husband's, my mother was diabetic and died of a heart attack at 93. She was a

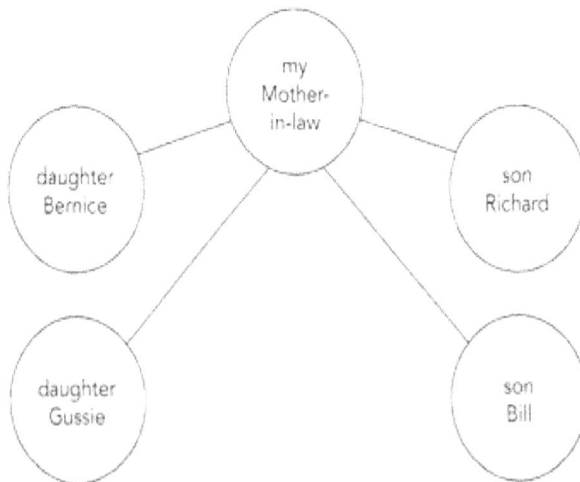

to delay or prevent diabetes. All along the way I kept hearing that fat around the waist and "belly fat" are the most dangerous. The fat puts strain on the heart to get blood to the lower extremities. And also tends to "strangle" other abdominal organs, making them less efficient. Most of all, fat interferes with proper insulin use by the cells for energy.

Research has shown that obese people, who are not diabetic,

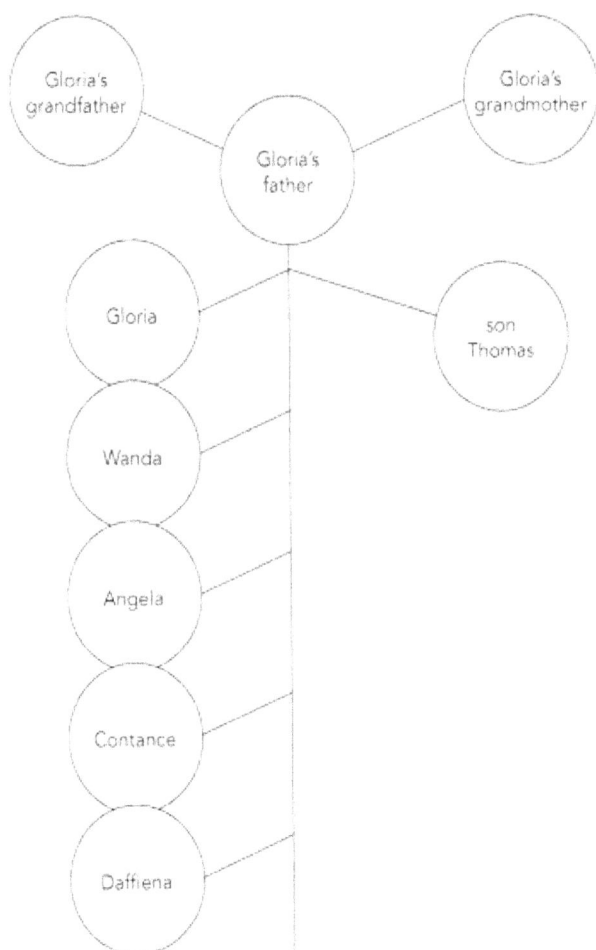

suffered organ failure at about the same rate as people whose body mass index was at a healthy level. But people with diabetes, no matter their weight, were three times more likely to suffer acute organ failure, and three times more likely to die from any cause than people who did not have diabetes.

Confounding to me at this point was how all the "plump" women in my Mississippi community neither died of diabetes per se, nor were there any messages about losing weight. Overweight was the norm. Nobody was weight-conscious. But my colleagues say everybody walked where they were going and had access to fresh vegetables, fruit and meat.

I would like to share with you my first experience with diabetes, which came after high school graduation. I was at my second job in Des Moines, Iowa, at Johnson's Nursing Home as a "practical nurse." I had no license, knowledge or training about diabetes. One of my high school teachers had encouraged me to "be a nurse, if not a teacher." I thought this job was a good start.

I assure you that it is not one of my proudest memories. Since then, the hundreds of nursing students to whom I taught insulin administration have heard my story due to its importance and impact. For several days I was given an orientation to the facility to learn the routine, then one day left on my own, self-assured that I could manage the work. And besides, I needed a job.

The patient was to get his insulin injection before he ate his breakfast. Mary, the kitchen person, notified me that Mr. Bingham's breakfast was ready. I had prepared the injection, and gave it to him. When Mary went back to help Mr. Bingham with his breakfast, he had classic symptoms of insulin overdose. She quickly went into action and counteracted the overdose of insulin with sugar and orange juice. He had no residual effects, but Mary called Mrs. Johnson, the director and owner. Evidently, Mr. Bingham had been stabilized on his diabetic regime, until I gave the insulin. So, when Mrs. Johnson inquired about his insulin that morning, it never occurred to me that

I gave him too much.

Things had gone okay for several days. I drew up the insulin, and gave it to Mr. Bingham. Mary fed him. On the day of the incident I had broken the only insulin syringe we had. The patient needed his insulin, before he could eat. But instead of calling Mrs. Johnson, I reasoned that if that amount of insulin in the insulin syringe was correct, then this amount in a 2 cc syringe would be the right amount. The worst part of the incident was I was not aware of having done wrong, until Mrs. Johnson did her investigation.

"Only give insulin with an i-n-s-u-l-i-n syringe," she said.

In summary, excess body fat does impact diabetes Type II, causing insulin resistance. However, the incidence is greater for getting the disease if it is in one's genes and the person becomes obese.

The symptoms of Diabetes Type II include the following:
• Frequent urination
• Excessive thirst or hunger
• Increased appetite
• Unexplained weight loss ·
• Blurry vision
• Fatigue
• Abdominal pain
• Nausea and/or vomiting
• Slow-healing sores
• Cramps or numbness in legs, feet or fingers
• Dry mouth
• Nervousness and/or dry, itchy skin
• No symptoms (testing needed to confirm)

Diabetes Type II develops gradually and usually affects those who are overweight or obese and over 40 years of age.

.

CHAPTER 3

We Are What We Eat

*Sometimes the hardest goal of all
can be changing the way we eat.*

-Fabiola D. Gaines, RD, LD
-Roniece Weaver, MS, RD, LD
American Diabetes Association

I FIRMLY AGREE WITH THE QUOTE ABOVE!

Many years ago Peg Bracken wrote the popular book, *I Hate to Cook*. Since cooking does not actually thrill me, my title would have been, I Love to Eat. For me, eating is enjoyable. However, my meals do not exactly help my overweight problem. Eating out with friends is pure enjoyment and I do like my own cooking and generally what others cook, too.

So, in simple terms, my problem with obesity mainly dealt with my relationship to food in many ways. One of the most important problems that faced me was that the food consumed required more attention and, as well, it was now my job to make various decisions about the food: The questions: How much? How often? Difficult decisions had to be made. Clearly, the basic need was to change my inner thoughts about managing the food.

Being morbidly obese, my immediate goal was to get under 200 pounds without going on a "quick-fix" diet or having surgery. Knowing that the pounds would return more quickly than they left, I decided to make a lifestyle change about food...and eating. Pamela

Lee, a UCLA dietitian helped me with my plan.

At the time I started the weight reduction program with Pamela, she provided me with a revised Food Guide Pyramid of the foods to include in my diet and the amounts. Then in June, 2011 the USDA changed the Pyramid as the guide, now using a visual representation called, My Plate, to simplify healthy eating.

According to Pamela the biggest difference between the original Food Guide Pyramid and the current My Plate is the emphasis on a larger amount of vegetables in the diet. In addition, the dietary guidelines for My Plate suggests: Eating more fruits, whole grains and fat-free or 1% milk and dairy products; choose foods with lower sodium content; and drink water instead of sugary drinks.

Since the changes to the Food Guide Pyramid were minor, Pamela initially suggested that serving size works better for me than counting calories.

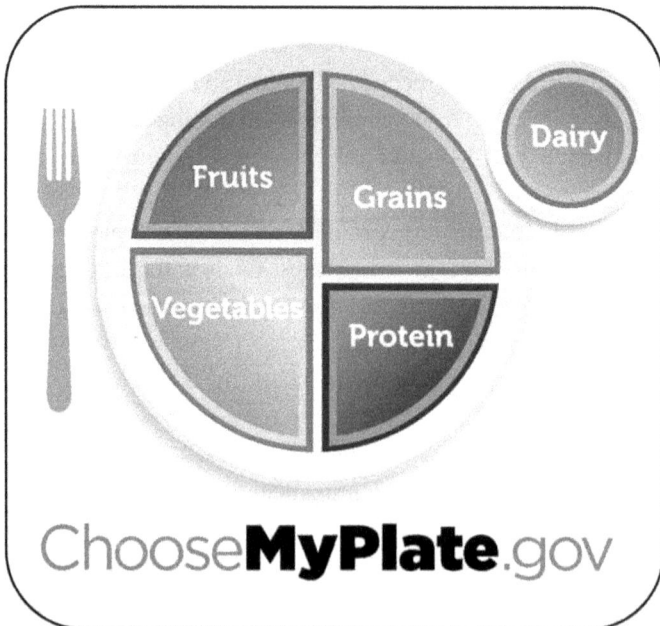

Pamela's Nutrition Guide

WHAT COUNTS AS ONE SERVING?

Fruit Group

1 piece or 1/2 cup of most fruits
1/2 banana
1 cup melon or berries
2 T dried fruit
1/2 cup juice

4 servings per day

Vegetable Group

1/2 cup chopped vegetables 1 cup leafy vegetables
4+ servings (unlimited)

Whole Grain and Beans Group

1 slice whole-grain bread
1/3 cup cooked whole grains (brown rice)
1/2 cup cooked whole-grain cereal (oatmeal)
3/4 cup whole-grain, ready-to-eat cereal (Cheerios)
1/2 cup beans and lentils
1/2 cup popcorn, peas and sweet potato

4 servings per day

Oils, Nuts and Seeds Group

1 T oil, 1 T salad dressing
1 T nuts or seeds (1/4 cup nuts-4 servings)
1/8 avocado
1/2 T peanut butter

3-6 servings per day

Low-fat Dairy Group

1 cup milk or yogurt
1 oz. cheese
1/4 cup soft or shredded cheese
1/2 cup cottage cheese

2 servings per day

Fish, Chicken and Soy Foods Group

3 oz. fish, poultry and soy analogues or lean meat
Count 1 egg as 1/2 serving

2 servings per day

Sweets, Saturated Fats, Etc.

This food group includes chips and alcohol.
Limit these foods to small amounts. What size portion do you need to satisfy?

Pamela's Notes to Me

• Ask for double veggies when eating out and put 1/2 of the meal in a "to go box.'
• Eat only when hungry.
• Stop before full.
• Serve yourself 1/3 less food: wait 15 minutes before having more food.
• Exercise, dancing thirty minutes, going to Curves, or walking 30 minutes 3-4 days a week.
• Keep a food diary.
• Follow meal plan.
• Watch the bread basket at restaurants. Take a little and ask server to remove it. Eat one small roll or ten chips.

Goals from Pamela

• **Goals**

1)   Exercise - Walk or gym workout 45 minutes, 4-6 days per week
2)   Food diary
3) Work towards the above two goals over the long term.
My Response
The food diary is an invaluable tool in anyone's weight-loss effort and it works for me. Write it down. You will not regret it.
Sometimes one hears what one wants to hear rather than what was said.

Pamela's Notes on
Quick and Easy Foods for Busy People

Below are some suggestions for fast, healthy meals and snacks. These recommendations balance carbohydrate and protein, are low in saturated fats, and provide lots of needed vitamins, minerals, and fiber.

Breakfast

Probably the most important meal of the day, breakfast is often skipped or eaten "on the run." Try some of these suggestions to start your day.

- Eggs and whole-grain toast. (Hard-boil eggs in advance and store in refrigerator.)
- Cottage cheese and fruit.
- Whole-grain toast with peanut butter or low-fat cheese.
- Whole-grain toaster waffles with peanut butter and a small amount of jam.
- Whole-grain toast with low-fat frozen sausage or Canadian bacon.
- Cereal and low-fat milk or yogurt, or low-fat string cheese.
- Apple or banana with peanut butter or low-fat cheese.
- Oatmeal with half cup berries.

Lunch

- An important meal for mid-day refueling. Below are some foods which can be prepared the night before and brown-bagged for a tasty meal.
- Turkey sandwich made with packaged sliced turkey breast.
- Tuna sandwich made with low-fat mayonnaise (try adding some lettuce, tomato, or other vegetables to sandwiches).
- Pre-washed bagged salad mix with water-packed canned tuna. Use a low-fat dressing or try olive oil and balsamic vinegar, and Italian seasoning.
- Peanut butter and jelly sandwich (use a small amount of jelly).
- Broth-based chicken soups.
- Frozen low-fat meals.

Dinner

The heaviest meal of the day for most people. Respond to your hunger throughout the day so dinner can be a light, nutritious meal.

- Pre-cooked roasted chicken with vegetables. (Pre-cooked roasted chickens are available at most supermarkets.)

.

- Baked potato with cottage cheese and frozen broccoli.
- Tuna melt - water-packed canned tuna and low-fat shredded cheese on whole grain bread.
- Bean and cheese burrito (use canned beans and low-fat Shredded cheese).
- Frozen veggie burger on small bun.
- Pre-washed bagged salad mix with sliced packaged turkey breast, and other pre-cut vegetables, canned mandarin orange slices, canned garbanzo beans and slivered almonds. Use a low- fat dressing or try olive oil and balsamic vinegar.

Snacks

Vital to a healthy meal plan. Try some of these super snacks when you start to feel a little hungry.

- Whole-grain crackers with low-fat cheese or peanut butter.
- Pre-cut raw vegetables and bean dip.
- Fruit and string cheese.
- Low-fat yogurt with sunflower seeds.
- Hard-boiled egg and an orange.
- Celery, carrots, apple or banana with peanut butter.
- Trail mix dried fruit and nuts.

Dining Out

Plan Ahead

- Choose a restaurant with a varied menu.
- Decide what type of food you will eat ahead of time.
- Plan other daily meals around your dining out choice.
- Don't arrive famished!

Control Portions

- Ask for a doggy bag at the beginning of the meal.
- Share your portion with a friend.
- Drink water, six to eight glasses daily.
- Order à la carte.
- Choose an appetizer as a main dish.

- Think small: half sandwich, cup of soup.
- Proceed with caution to buffets and smorgasbords. Limit these restaurants.

Decrease Fat

- Be assertive. Ask questions about food preparation.
- Order chicken, fish, or pasta marinara dishes.
- Limit fried foods.
- Limit foods with butter, cream, or cheese sauces.
- Choose baked, broiled, grilled, steamed, roasted foods.
- Ask for salad dressing, margarine, and sour cream on the side.
- Avoid mayonnaise-based salads such as tuna, potato, and coleslaw.
- Choose fresh fruit or sherbet or flavored coffees for dessert.
- Learn to read food labels:

Food Label Decoder

SERVING SIZE

Check to see if your serving is the same size as the one on the label. If you eat double the serving size listed, you need to double the nutrient and caloric values. If you eat one-half the serving size shown here, the nutrient and caloric values should be halved.

CALORIES

Look here to see what a serving of food adds to your daily total. A person's size and activity level help determine total calories needed per day. For example, a 138-lb active woman needs about 2,000 calories each day, while a 160-lb active woman needs about 2,300.

TOTAL CARBOHYDRATES

Carbohydrates are found in foods such as bread, potatoes, fruits, milk, vegetables, and sweets. Carbohydrates are the main source of energy for body functions. Talk to your healthcare provider/dietitian about the amount of carbohydrates to have in your meal plan.

DIETARY FIBER

It is important to consume foods containing fiber from a wide variety of sources. Fruits, vegetables, whole-grain foods, beans, and legumes are all good sources of fiber and can help lower cholesterol and thus reduce the risk of heart disease. Consumption of 20-35 grams per day is generally recommended.

SUGARS

Labels will indicate the grams of sugars in a food-both the natural and the added sugars. Since sugars are a type of carbohydrate, the most important number to look at on the label is the total amount of carbohydrates for the serving you are eating. Talk to your healthcare provider/dietitian about the use of sugar to have in your meal plan.

VITAMINS AND MINERALS

Make it your goal to get 100% of each every day. Let a combination of foods contribute to a winning score.

Nutrition Facts

Serving Size 2 tortillas (51g)
Servings Per Container 6

Amount Per Serving

Calories 110   Calories from Fat 10

                        %Daily Value*

Total Fat 1g	**2%**
Saturated Fat 0g	**0%**
Trans Fat 0g	
Cholesterol 0mg	**0%**
Sodium 30mg	**1%**
Total Carbohydrate 22g	**7%**
Dietary Fiber 2g	**8%**
Sugars 0g	
Protein 2g	

Vitamin A 0%		Vitamin C 0%	
Calcium 2%		Iron 4%	

* Percent Daily Values are based on a 2,000 calorie diet. Your Daily Values may be higher or lower depending on your calorie needs.

	Calories	2,000	2,500
Total Fat	Less than	65g	80g
Sat Fat	Less than	20g	25g
Cholesterol	Less than	300mg	300mg
Sodium	Less than	2,400mg	2,400mg
Total Carb		300g	375g
Dietary Fiber		25g	30g

TOTAL FAT

Try to limit your calories from fat. Too much fat may contribute to heart disease and cancer. Choose foods with less than 30% of calories derived from fat.

SATURATED FAT

Saturated fat is the "bad" fat. It is the key player in raising blood cholesterol and your risk of heart disease. Less than 10% of daily calories should come from saturated fat.

CHOLESTEROL

Challenge yourself to eat foods totaling less than 300 mg of cholesterol a day. Too much cholesterol can lead to heart disease. Cholesterol is found in foods of animal origin, such as meat, fish, eggs, and whole-milk products such as cheese and butter. Certain food products that contain plant stanols/sterols (for example, cholesterol-lowering margarine) can also help lower cholesterol.

SODIUM

Too much sodium (or salt) adds up to high blood pressure in some people. Sodium intake should be 2,400 mg per day, or even lower depending on your health. Talk to your healthcare provider/dietitian about the amount of sodium to have in your diet.

PROTEIN

Most adults get more protein than they need. Even though protein from animal sources such as meat, fish, milk, and cheese is of higher nutritional quality than plant-based protein, it is also higher in fat - especially saturated fat and cholesterol. Use skim or low-fat milk, yogurt, and cheese. Try to get some protein from vegetables (such as beans, grains, and cereals).

DAILY VALUES

These daily values apply to people who eat 2,000 to 2,500 calories each day. If you eat less, your personal daily value may be lower.

Additional nutrients may be listed on some food labels.
g = grams (about 28 g = 1 ounce), mg = milligrams (1,000 mg = 1 g)

Food Suggestions
Ethnic Low-fat Food Choices

ETHNICITY	CHOOSE MORE OFTEN	CHOOSE LESS OFTEN
CHINESE	• Steamed or lightly stir-fried chicken, lean meat, rice or vegetables. • Mix one cup entrée with one cup steamed rice or steamed vegetables to dilute the sauce.	• Fried entrees, fried rice, fried wonton, fried noodles • Egg roll • Peking duck • Pork, spare ribs
ITALIAN	• Pasta with Marinara Sauce. • Vegetarian pizza with little or no cheese.	• Pasta with butter, cream, Alfredo, cheese, meat and pesto sauce • Lasagna, eggplant, or veal Parmesan • Caesar salad • Sausage, pepperoni, or cheese pizza
MEXICAN	• Chicken, fish, lean meat, beans and vegetables cooked without adding oil • Bean burrito or enchilada without cheese • Salsa • Corn tortillas	• Regular burritos, tacos, enchiladas • Chile rellenos • Refried beans • Guacamole and sour cream • Cheese • Corn chips • Nachos

SOUTHERN COUSINE	<ul><li>Baked chicken, fish, potatoes, boiled greens, blacked-eyed peas, sweet potatoes, beans (all cooked without ham hock – substitute turkey)</li><li>Grits without butter and cheese</li><li>Gumbo and Jambalaya cooked with lean meats and limited salt</li><li>Blackened fish</li></ul>	<ul><li>Fried chicken, fish, and potatoes</li><li>Ham, bacon, sausage</li><li>Chitlins</li><li>Cornbread, biscuits</li><li>Fried alligator</li><li>Peach cobber</li><li>Butter pound cake</li></ul>
JAPANESE	<ul><li>Grilled chicken, fish or lean meat</li><li>Sushi, sashimi</li></ul>	<ul><li>Tempura</li><li>Teriyaki beef</li></ul>

With all this information at my fingertips it was time to plan for my successful food management and lifestyle change. I understood that the first day in the process would be my hardest because I had traveled that road before and also knew that as the stomach adjusts to having less food in it, it will shrink. So the urge to eat large portions will diminish over time. Plan the first day well and the following days will become easier.

Keep in mind the old proverb: "If you can do something for twenty-one days, it becomes a habit." I asked myself what better habit is more important than a lifestyle change to reduce my weight and possibly prevent or delay the onset of diabetes. While we tire of specific diets, we never tire of food. We can always change our choices and that makes it interesting as well as challenging.

I found that a diary:

- Keeps me on track.
- Provides a record.
- Allows me to remember when and what was eaten.
- Maintains accuracy.
- Provides the painful awareness that morsels also have calories.
- And, most of all, helps to develop a good habit.

My success has been better with the staying power of exercise than with diet. It was never a consideration about abandoning my goal of being free of diabetes. My guilt lies in mindless eating, backsliding and frustration upon reaching a plateau.

Simply said, mindless eating occurs, when we eat without thinking about *what* we are eating, *how much or how fattening* the food is. This sort of eating is temporary. Disappointment comes with the realization of the necessity for me to ask: What have I done? The lesson learned is to keep low-calorie foods in my house.

Backsliding can be more long-term, say, a day or several days. Social activities require my presence, leaving me no time to prepare what I eat. Again, the lesson here: be selective.

The plateau is the most frustrating because downward weight

movement seems impossible sometimes. I have to cut back on the amount of food consumed, not including protein. I vary the form of exercise with a slight increase in time performed. I shun added salt, drink lots of water and get 7-1/2 to 8 hours of sleep. I find this doable.

Whatever you decide about your weight or weight problems, try to avoid my friend's attitude.

As though I have a magic wand, my obese friend has told me for more than several months that she needs to lose weight. The problem is that she is a "couch potato" who enjoys trying recipes she sees on TV. Walking and other forms of exercise are not her strong suit. Most recently she said, "I can't lose any weight, so I am going to stop trying."

Long before she reaches staying power she needs short-term willpower, such as getting off the couch more and preparing healthier dishes.

Pamela Lee reminded me again and I remind you: "Eat only when you are hungry. And eat only enough to satisfy the hunger. Remember, it takes twenty minutes for the brain to get the message that you are no longer hungry."

In summary, we know that there was an obesity problem with me. Not only is obesity a problem in itself but it tends to cause many other health problems, diabetes type II being one of them, especially if there is an inherited tendency.

Following a serving size list, I have prepared a food diary for you to fill out each day for twenty-one days. Try to stick with it. Should you "fall off the wagon," start back as soon as you can. The next time, try to avoid the reason(s) that caused the problem the last time.

SERVING SIZE

PROTEIN

(Measure raw, uncooked unless otherwise noted)
Lindora Protein products, variety
Beef heart, ground, 3-1/2 oz.
Beef flank, 3-1/2 oz.
Beef sirloin, lean ground, 3 oz.
Beef round, 3-1/2 oz.
Chicken breast, 3-1/2 oz.
Chicken breast, canned 2-1/2 oz.
Cold cuts, 98% fat-free, 2-1/2 oz.
Pork tenderloin, lean, 3 oz.
Turkey, white breast, 3-1/2 oz.
Turkey breast, ground, 97% lean, 3-12 oz. Veal, 3-1/2 oz.
Cheese, fat-free, 2 oz.
Cottage cheese, low-fat, 4 oz.
Egg, whole, 1
Egg whites, 2
Milk, non-fat, 1 c
Yogurt, plain fat-free, 1/2 c
Tofu, low-fat, 6 oz.
Veggie burger, low-fat
Catfish, 3-1/2 oz.
Cod, 3-1/2 oz.
Crab, 3-1/2 oz.
Haddock, 3-1/2 oz.
Halibut, 3-1/2 oz.
Lobster, 3-1/2 oz.
Orange Roughy, 3-1/2 oz.
Perch, 3-1/2 oz.
Salmon, 3-1/2 oz.

Scallops, 3-1/2 oz.
Sea bass, 3-1/2 oz.
Shark, 3-1/2 oz.
Shrimp, 3-1/2 oz.
Snapper, 3-1/2 oz.
Sole, 3-1/2 oz.
Swordfish, 3-1/2 oz.
Trout, rainbow, 3-1/2 oz.
Tuna, fresh or frozen, 2-1/2 oz.
Tuna, canned in water, 2-1/2 oz.
Turbot, 3-1/2 oz.

GRAINS
(Choice of one serving of fruit OR grain, at breakfast)
Bread, whole-grain, 1 slice, 80 calories or less
Cream of Wheat, cooked, 1/2 c
Cream of Rice, cooked, 1/2 c
Oatmeal, cooked, 1/2 c
Cereal, dry, variety, 1/2 - 3/4 c 80 - 110 calories

VEGETABLES
(Measure uncooked unless otherwise noted)
Asparagus, 1 c
Bean sprouts, 1 c
Broccoli, 1 c
Cabbage, 1 c
Carrots, 1/2 c
Celery, 1 c
Chinese pea pods, 1 c
Cauliflower, 1 c
Collard greens, 1 c
Cucumbers, 1 c Jicama, 1/2 c

Mushrooms, raw, 2 c
Okra, 1 c
Onion, 1/2 c
Pepper, red or green, 1 sm
Spinach, raw, 2 c
Spinach, cooked, 1 c
String beans, 1 c
Sauerkraut, 1 c
Tomato, 1 sm
Zucchini, 1 c

FRUITS
Apple, 2-1/2"
Applesauce, unsw, 1/2 c
Apricots, fresh, 2 med
Apricots, dried, 4 halves
Banana, 1/2 sm
Blackberries, 2/3 c
Blueberries, 2/3 c
Boysenberries, 2/3 c
Casaba melon, 1/4 sm
Cantaloupe, 1/4 sm
Cherries, 10
Dates, 2
Grapefruit, 1/2 sm
Grapefruit juice, unsweet
Honeydew melon, 1/6 sm Kiwi, 3 oz.
Nectarine, 1/2 c sliced
Orange, 1 sm (14)
Orange juice, unsweet, 1/2 c
Papaya, 1/2 c cubed
Peach, 1 sm

Pear (Bartlett), 1/2 sm
Persimmon, 1
Pineapple, 1/2 c cubed
Raisins, 1/2 oz.
Raspberries, 2/3 c
Rhubarb, 1 c
Strawberries, 1 c
Tangerine, 2-1/2"
Watermelon, 1/2 c cubed

MISCELLANEOUS
(One serving, twice a day with meal)
Coffee creamer, powder, 1 tsp.
Gelatin, sugar-free, 1/2 c
Green onion, tops, 1 tsp.
Horseradish, 1 tsp.
Margarine, fat-free, 1 Tbsp.
Mustard, 1 tsp.
Jalapeno peppers, 2 sm
Pimento, 2 sm
Radishes, 2 med
Vinegar, 2 T

(Make It a Habit)
Day 1
My 21-Day, Don't Call It a Diet Diary

Day: _____

Vitamin _____ Glasses of water _____ Minutes of Exercise _____ Weight _____

Time	Nutrition Plan	Serving Size	Satisfied?
_____	Breakfast		
	Protein	_____	_____
	Fruit or Grain	_____	_____
	Beverage	_____	_____
_____	Snack	_____	_____
_____	Lunch		
	Protein	_____	_____
	Vegetable	_____	_____
	Lettuce	_____	_____
	Fruit	_____	_____
	Beverage	_____	_____
	Miscellaneous	_____	_____
_____	Snack	_____	_____
_____	Dinner		
	Protein	_____	_____
	Vegetable	_____	_____
	Lettuce	_____	_____
	Fruit	_____	_____
	Beverage	_____	_____
	Miscellaneous	_____	_____
_____	Snack	_____	_____

(Make It a Habit)
Day 2
My 21-Day, Don't Call It a Diet Diary

Day: _____

Vitamin _____ Glasses of water _____ Minutes of Exercise _____ Weight _____

Time	Nutrition Plan	Serving Size	Satisfied?
_____	Breakfast		
	Protein	_____	_____
	Fruit or Grain	_____	_____
	Beverage	_____	_____
_____	Snack	_____	_____
_____	Lunch		
	Protein	_____	_____
	Vegetable	_____	_____
	Lettuce	_____	_____
	Fruit	_____	_____
	Beverage	_____	_____
	Miscellaneous	_____	_____
_____	Snack	_____	_____
_____	Dinner		
	Protein	_____	_____
	Vegetable	_____	_____
	Lettuce	_____	_____
	Fruit	_____	_____
	Beverage	_____	_____
	Miscellaneous	_____	_____
_____	Snack	_____	_____

(Make It a Habit)
Day 3
My 21-Day, Don't Call It a Diet Diary

Day: _____

Vitamin _____ Glasses of water _____Minutes of Exercise _____ Weight _____

Time	Nutrition Plan	Serving Size	Satisfied?
_____	Breakfast		
	Protein	_____	_____
	Fruit or Grain	_____	_____
	Beverage	_____	_____
_____	Snack	_____	_____
_____	Lunch		
	Protein	_____	_____
	Vegetable	_____	_____
	Lettuce	_____	_____
	Fruit	_____	_____
	Beverage	_____	_____
	Miscellaneous	_____	_____
_____	Snack	_____	_____
_____	Dinner		
	Protein	_____	_____
	Vegetable	_____	_____
	Lettuce	_____	_____
	Fruit	_____	_____
	Beverage	_____	_____
	Miscellaneous	_____	_____
_____	Snack	_____	_____

(Make It a Habit)
Day 4
My 21-Day, Don't Call It a Diet Diary

Day: _____

Vitamin _____ Glasses of water _____ Minutes of Exercise _____ Weight _____

Time	Nutrition Plan	Serving Size	Satisfied?
_____	Breakfast Protein Fruit or Grain Beverage	 _____ _____ _____	 _____ _____ _____
_____	Snack	_____	_____
_____	Lunch Protein Vegetable Lettuce Fruit Beverage Miscellaneous	 _____ _____ _____ _____ _____ _____	 _____ _____ _____ _____ _____ _____
_____	Snack	_____	_____
_____	Dinner Protein Vegetable Lettuce Fruit Beverage Miscellaneous	 _____ _____ _____ _____ _____ _____	 _____ _____ _____ _____ _____ _____
_____	Snack	_____	_____

(Make It a Habit)
Day 5
My 21-Day, Don't Call It a Diet Diary

Day: _____

Vitamin _____ Glasses of water _____Minutes of Exercise _____ Weight _____

Time	Nutrition Plan	Serving Size	Satisfied?
_____	Breakfast		
	Protein	_____	_____
	Fruit or Grain	_____	_____
	Beverage	_____	_____
_____	Snack	_____	_____
_____	Lunch		
	Protein	_____	_____
	Vegetable	_____	_____
	Lettuce	_____	_____
	Fruit	_____	_____
	Beverage	_____	_____
	Miscellaneous	_____	_____
_____	Snack	_____	_____
_____	Dinner		
	Protein	_____	_____
	Vegetable	_____	_____
	Lettuce	_____	_____
	Fruit	_____	_____
	Beverage	_____	_____
	Miscellaneous	_____	_____
_____	Snack	_____	_____

(Make It a Habit)
Day 6
My 21-Day, Don't Call It a Diet Diary

Day: _____

Vitamin _____ Glasses of water _____ Minutes of Exercise _____ Weight _____

Time	Nutrition Plan	Serving Size	Satisfied?
_____	Breakfast		
	Protein	_____	_____
	Fruit or Grain	_____	_____
	Beverage	_____	_____
_____	Snack	_____	_____
_____	Lunch		
	Protein	_____	_____
	Vegetable	_____	_____
	Lettuce	_____	_____
	Fruit	_____	_____
	Beverage	_____	_____
	Miscellaneous	_____	_____
_____	Snack	_____	_____
_____	Dinner		
	Protein	_____	_____
	Vegetable	_____	_____
	Lettuce	_____	_____
	Fruit	_____	_____
	Beverage	_____	_____
	Miscellaneous	_____	_____
_____	Snack	_____	_____

(Make It a Habit)
Day 7
My 21-Day, Don't Call It a Diet Diary

Day: _____

Vitamin _____ Glasses of water _____ Minutes of Exercise _____ Weight _____

Time	Nutrition Plan	Serving Size	Satisfied?
_____	Breakfast		
	Protein	_____	_____
	Fruit or Grain	_____	_____
	Beverage	_____	_____
_____	Snack	_____	_____
_____	Lunch		
	Protein	_____	_____
	Vegetable	_____	_____
	Lettuce	_____	_____
	Fruit	_____	_____
	Beverage	_____	_____
	Miscellaneous	_____	_____
_____	Snack	_____	_____
_____	Dinner		
	Protein	_____	_____
	Vegetable	_____	_____
	Lettuce	_____	_____
	Fruit	_____	_____
	Beverage	_____	_____
	Miscellaneous	_____	_____
_____	Snack	_____	_____

(Make It a Habit)
Day 8
My 21-Day, Don't Call It a Diet Diary

Day: _____

Vitamin _____ Glasses of water _____ Minutes of Exercise _____ Weight _____

Time	Nutrition Plan	Serving Size	Satisfied?
_____	Breakfast		
	Protein	_____	_____
	Fruit or Grain	_____	_____
	Beverage	_____	_____
_____	Snack	_____	_____
_____	Lunch		
	Protein	_____	_____
	Vegetable	_____	_____
	Lettuce	_____	_____
	Fruit	_____	_____
	Beverage	_____	_____
	Miscellaneous	_____	_____
_____	Snack	_____	_____
_____	Dinner		
	Protein	_____	_____
	Vegetable	_____	_____
	Lettuce	_____	_____
	Fruit	_____	_____
	Beverage	_____	_____
	Miscellaneous	_____	_____
_____	Snack	_____	_____

(Make It a Habit)
Day 9
My 21-Day, Don't Call It a Diet Diary

Day: _____

Vitamin _____ Glasses of water _____ Minutes of Exercise _____ Weight _____

Time	Nutrition Plan	Serving Size	Satisfied?
_____	Breakfast		
	Protein	_____	_____
	Fruit or Grain	_____	_____
	Beverage	_____	_____
_____	Snack	_____	_____
_____	Lunch		
	Protein	_____	_____
	Vegetable	_____	_____
	Lettuce	_____	_____
	Fruit	_____	_____
	Beverage	_____	_____
	Miscellaneous	_____	_____
_____	Snack	_____	_____
_____	Dinner		
	Protein	_____	_____
	Vegetable	_____	_____
	Lettuce	_____	_____
	Fruit	_____	_____
	Beverage	_____	_____
	Miscellaneous	_____	_____
_____	Snack	_____	_____

(Make It a Habit)
Day 10
My 21-Day, Don't Call It a Diet Diary

Day: _____

Vitamin _____ Glasses of water _____ Minutes of Exercise _____ Weight _____

Time	Nutrition Plan	Serving Size	Satisfied?
_____	Breakfast Protein Fruit or Grain Beverage	 _____ _____ _____	 _____ _____ _____
_____	Snack	_____	_____
_____	Lunch Protein Vegetable Lettuce Fruit Beverage Miscellaneous	 _____ _____ _____ _____ _____ _____	 _____ _____ _____ _____ _____ _____
_____	Snack	_____	_____
_____	Dinner Protein Vegetable Lettuce Fruit Beverage Miscellaneous	 _____ _____ _____ _____ _____ _____	 _____ _____ _____ _____ _____ _____
_____	Snack	_____	_____

(Make It a Habit)
Day 11
My 21-Day, Don't Call It a Diet Diary

Day: _____

Vitamin _____ Glasses of water _____ Minutes of Exercise _____ Weight _____

Time	Nutrition Plan	Serving Size	Satisfied?
_____	Breakfast		
	Protein	_____	_____
	Fruit or Grain	_____	_____
	Beverage	_____	_____
_____	Snack	_____	_____
_____	Lunch		
	Protein	_____	_____
	Vegetable	_____	_____
	Lettuce	_____	_____
	Fruit	_____	_____
	Beverage	_____	_____
	Miscellaneous	_____	_____
_____	Snack	_____	_____
_____	Dinner		
	Protein	_____	_____
	Vegetable	_____	_____
	Lettuce	_____	_____
	Fruit	_____	_____
	Beverage	_____	_____
	Miscellaneous	_____	_____
_____	Snack	_____	_____

(Make It a Habit)
Day 12
My 21-Day, Don't Call It a Diet Diary

Day: _____

Vitamin _____ Glasses of water _____ Minutes of Exercise _____ Weight _____

Time	Nutrition Plan	Serving Size	Satisfied?
_____	Breakfast		
	Protein	_____	_____
	Fruit or Grain	_____	_____
	Beverage	_____	_____
_____	Snack	_____	_____
_____	Lunch		
	Protein	_____	_____
	Vegetable	_____	_____
	Lettuce	_____	_____
	Fruit	_____	_____
	Beverage	_____	_____
	Miscellaneous	_____	_____
_____	Snack	_____	_____
_____	Dinner		
	Protein	_____	_____
	Vegetable	_____	_____
	Lettuce	_____	_____
	Fruit	_____	_____
	Beverage	_____	_____
	Miscellaneous	_____	_____
_____	Snack	_____	_____

(Make It a Habit)
Day 13
My 21-Day, Don't Call It a Diet Diary

Day: _____

Vitamin _____ Glasses of water _____ Minutes of Exercise _____ Weight _____

Time	Nutrition Plan	Serving Size	Satisfied?
_____	Breakfast Protein Fruit or Grain Beverage	 _____ _____ _____	 _____ _____ _____
_____	Snack	_____	_____
_____	Lunch Protein Vegetable Lettuce Fruit Beverage Miscellaneous	 _____ _____ _____ _____ _____ _____	 _____ _____ _____ _____ _____ _____
_____	Snack	_____	_____
_____	Dinner Protein Vegetable Lettuce Fruit Beverage Miscellaneous	 _____ _____ _____ _____ _____ _____	 _____ _____ _____ _____ _____ _____
_____	Snack	_____	_____

(Make It a Habit)
Day 14
My 21-Day, Don't Call It a Diet Diary

Day: _____

Vitamin _____ Glasses of water _____ Minutes of Exercise _____ Weight _____

Time	Nutrition Plan	Serving Size	Satisfied?
_____	Breakfast		
	Protein	_____	_____
	Fruit or Grain	_____	_____
	Beverage	_____	_____
_____	Snack	_____	_____
_____	Lunch		
	Protein	_____	_____
	Vegetable	_____	_____
	Lettuce	_____	_____
	Fruit	_____	_____
	Beverage	_____	_____
	Miscellaneous	_____	_____
_____	Snack	_____	_____
_____	Dinner		
	Protein	_____	_____
	Vegetable	_____	_____
	Lettuce	_____	_____
	Fruit	_____	_____
	Beverage	_____	_____
	Miscellaneous	_____	_____
_____	Snack	_____	_____

(Make It a Habit)
Day 15
My 21-Day, Don't Call It a Diet Diary

Day: _____

Vitamin _____ Glasses of water _____ Minutes of Exercise _____ Weight _____

Time	Nutrition Plan	Serving Size	Satisfied?
_____	Breakfast Protein Fruit or Grain Beverage	 _____ _____ _____	 _____ _____ _____
_____	Snack	_____	_____
_____	Lunch Protein Vegetable Lettuce Fruit Beverage Miscellaneous	 _____ _____ _____ _____ _____ _____	 _____ _____ _____ _____ _____ _____
_____	Snack	_____	_____
_____	Dinner Protein Vegetable Lettuce Fruit Beverage Miscellaneous	 _____ _____ _____ _____ _____ _____	 _____ _____ _____ _____ _____ _____
_____	Snack	_____	_____

(Make It a Habit)
Day 16
My 21-Day, Don't Call It a Diet Diary

Day: _____

Vitamin _____ Glasses of water _____ Minutes of Exercise _____ Weight _____

Time	Nutrition Plan	Serving Size	Satisfied?
_____	Breakfast Protein Fruit or Grain Beverage	_____ _____ _____	_____ _____ _____
_____	Snack	_____	_____
_____	Lunch Protein Vegetable Lettuce Fruit Beverage Miscellaneous	_____ _____ _____ _____ _____ _____	_____ _____ _____ _____ _____ _____
_____	Snack	_____	_____
_____	Dinner Protein Vegetable Lettuce Fruit Beverage Miscellaneous	_____ _____ _____ _____ _____ _____	_____ _____ _____ _____ _____ _____
_____	Snack	_____	_____

(Make It a Habit)
Day 17
My 21-Day, Don't Call It a Diet Diary

Day: _____

Vitamin _____ Glasses of water _____Minutes of Exercise _____ Weight _____

Time	Nutrition Plan	Serving Size	Satisfied?
_____	Breakfast Protein Fruit or Grain Beverage	 _____ _____ _____	 _____ _____ _____
_____	Snack	_____	_____
_____	Lunch Protein Vegetable Lettuce Fruit Beverage Miscellaneous	 _____ _____ _____ _____ _____ _____	 _____ _____ _____ _____ _____ _____
_____	Snack	_____	_____
_____	Dinner Protein Vegetable Lettuce Fruit Beverage Miscellaneous	 _____ _____ _____ _____ _____ _____	 _____ _____ _____ _____ _____ _____
_____	Snack	_____	_____

(Make It a Habit)
Day 18
My 21-Day, Don't Call It a Diet Diary

Day: _____

Vitamin _____ Glasses of water _____ Minutes of Exercise _____ Weight _____

Time	Nutrition Plan	Serving Size	Satisfied?
_____	Breakfast		
	Protein	_____	_____
	Fruit or Grain	_____	_____
	Beverage	_____	_____
_____	Snack	_____	_____
_____	Lunch		
	Protein	_____	_____
	Vegetable	_____	_____
	Lettuce	_____	_____
	Fruit	_____	_____
	Beverage	_____	_____
	Miscellaneous	_____	_____
_____	Snack	_____	_____
_____	Dinner		
	Protein	_____	_____
	Vegetable	_____	_____
	Lettuce	_____	_____
	Fruit	_____	_____
	Beverage	_____	_____
	Miscellaneous	_____	_____
_____	Snack	_____	_____

(Make It a Habit)
Day 19
My 21-Day, Don't Call It a Diet Diary

Day: _____

Vitamin _____ Glasses of water _____Minutes of Exercise _____ Weight _____

Time	Nutrition Plan	Serving Size	Satisfied?
_____	Breakfast Protein Fruit or Grain Beverage	 _____ _____ _____	 _____ _____ _____
_____	Snack	_____	_____
_____	Lunch Protein Vegetable Lettuce Fruit Beverage Miscellaneous	 _____ _____ _____ _____ _____ _____	 _____ _____ _____ _____ _____ _____
_____	Snack	_____	_____
_____	Dinner Protein Vegetable Lettuce Fruit Beverage Miscellaneous	 _____ _____ _____ _____ _____ _____	 _____ _____ _____ _____ _____ _____
_____	Snack	_____	_____

(Make It a Habit)
Day 20
My 21-Day, Don't Call It a Diet Diary

Day: _____

Vitamin _____ Glasses of water _____Minutes of Exercise _____ Weight _____

Time	Nutrition Plan	Serving Size	Satisfied?
_____	Breakfast		
	Protein	_____	_____
	Fruit or Grain	_____	_____
	Beverage	_____	_____
_____	Snack	_____	_____
_____	Lunch		
	Protein	_____	_____
	Vegetable	_____	_____
	Lettuce	_____	_____
	Fruit	_____	_____
	Beverage	_____	_____
	Miscellaneous	_____	_____
_____	Snack	_____	_____
_____	Dinner		
	Protein	_____	_____
	Vegetable	_____	_____
	Lettuce	_____	_____
	Fruit	_____	_____
	Beverage	_____	_____
	Miscellaneous	_____	_____
_____	Snack	_____	_____

(Make It a Habit)
Day 21
My 21-Day, Don't Call It a Diet Diary

Day: _____

Vitamin _____ Glasses of water _____Minutes of Exercise _____ Weight _____

Time	Nutrition Plan	Serving Size	Satisfied?
_____	Breakfast		
	Protein	_____	_____
	Fruit or Grain	_____	_____
	Beverage	_____	_____
_____	Snack	_____	_____
_____	Lunch		
	Protein	_____	_____
	Vegetable	_____	_____
	Lettuce	_____	_____
	Fruit	_____	_____
	Beverage	_____	_____
	Miscellaneous	_____	_____
_____	Snack	_____	_____
_____	Dinner		
	Protein	_____	_____
	Vegetable	_____	_____
	Lettuce	_____	_____
	Fruit	_____	_____
	Beverage	_____	_____
	Miscellaneous	_____	_____
_____	Snack	_____	_____

Now, we know that the food we eat, as well as the amount, play important roles in treating both obesity and diabetes. Our next step is to examine the important role that exercise plays in the process of weight loss and diabetes prevention or delay.

CHAPTER 4

Exercise and Diet

The single most effective prescription
for reducing and treating disease is exercise.

- C. Noel Bairney Merz
Director of Women's Health
Cedars-Sinai Medical Center
Los Angeles

THE WORD "AWESOME" IS WHAT comes to mind as I reflect on all the new learning that I now possess. For the first time I am cognizant that exercise is a universal tonic for being healthy. My lifestyle has changed for the better, and exercise is now both an important as well as a fun aspect of living. I enjoy walking and working out as much as I do eating out.

Shortly after I completed the 2011 Los Angeles Marathon, I happened to be engaged in a lively conversation with a group of friends. At one point, I started to say, "When I went walking this morning..."

Very abruptly, one person said in a scolding voice, "Are you STILL walking?"

I chose to ignore the question, but felt disappointed that the friend did not have a clue about how important walking is to staying power for me. So let this incident be a reminder to you: Not everyone will support your fitness effort or understand why you are doing what you do or they may be just envious...

Since I started the weight-loss and physical fitness process to decrease my chances of getting diabetes, my knowledge of the relationship between metabolism and losing weight has increased two-fold. Other essential areas with weight loss include walking, the use of body weights and exercise in general. I also have a much better understanding of what occurs when the body reaches those dreaded weight-loss plateaus, a period where no apparent weight loss occurs with the same effort.

Although I was aware that aging slows the metabolic process, it is inexplicable to me why I never bothered to learn more about the body's mechanisms and metabolism until now. Metabolism is important to weight-loss efforts. Metabolism is defined as the rate at which the body burns calories. The higher the metabolic rate, the more calories are burned for a period of time and thus the greater the amount of weight loss.

The metabolic rate adjusts according to one's activity level. The rate is slower while one sleeps than if one is jogging or running fast. The length of time one is engaged in an activity, as well the intensity, also affect metabolism. For example, a brisk walk for five minutes is more intensive and beneficial to the heart and circulation than a casual walk for five minutes. According to Bob Greene (2002.67), you can bring more permanent changes to total metabolism and "elevate it all twenty-four hours each day of your life" by regular aerobic exercising. He further states that this is one of the secrets of making dramatically positive changes to your body.

Dr. Davis's face lit up when I told her of my plans for a summer trip to Washington, D.C., for my sorority's centennial celebration. We were planning my next blood-work appointment. She seemed excited, having recently visited the city during cherry blossom time to see her daughter. My appointment with Dr. Davis ended with advice given in her official role, "Do a lot of walking." She had not forgotten my eating habits, and a simple brisk walk could only help to prevent diabetes and enhances the body's ability to handle glucose.

Walking plays many roles in health: it enhances blood circulation, helps with the high blood pressure, and improves cholesterol level. All of these improvements are important in preventing diabetes, heart disease and obesity, which is a risk factor for all the above, as well as enhancing the brain's neurotransmitters for lifting depression, thus improving one's mood or creativity.

Walking produces great benefits with little fuss. Neither equipment nor any special training books are needed. Walking can be individualized according to need. Many times I walk with Cookie, my canine companion, and sometimes walk alone. Cookie has an attitude, when walking with me, so I enjoy my walking time alone. Invariably, there is an interesting plant, tree or pet that I had not seen before. I am never disappointed after walking, only from falling asleep on the couch watching TV or procrastinating about going.

Walking is apparently the exercise of choice among fitness experts and doctors. Walking as an exercise is easy on the joints, strengthens bones, and it helps to improve our well-being, coordination, speed and agility (Shapiro 2000.242). Most importantly for me, walking has prevented the onset of diabetes.

Be prepared, however, to make changes in your walking routine, as the body sometimes gets bored with the same routine and nothing happens weight-wise. You can do intervals of brisk walking during the regular walk, increase the length of time, go up hills or inclines, carrying light weights. I usually walk with a sauna belt (with ribs on it) for my stomach, mid-section and intra-abdominal fat.

Having reached a plateau with my walking program, Todd Burkholder, my exercise physiologist, suggested that I work out with weights. I promptly acquired membership at the local YMCA. For the first ten weeks I had a personal trainer to make sure I did not injure myself and now work out three times per week and like the results.

Although body weights are not associated with diabetes, in terms of osteoporosis, I was asked by my YMCA fitness chairperson to note that body weights workouts help bone to release calcium for muscle contraction. This form of activity helps prevent osteoporosis and is important for older women. Todd never explained that the weights were not cardio training, but build and strengthen muscles, which helps the body burn glucose more efficiently and utilize insulin better. I have been pleased with the results.

In no way should you be misled to believe that walking is the only recommended form of exercise. Although walking is probably the simplest, safest, and one of the most effective overall exercises for circulation, heart health, bones and well-being, do not neglect general exercises: dancing; swimming; water aerobics; indoor and outdoor cycling; fitness centers; treadmills; and gyms. Half an hour per day is usually recommended; 45 minutes or more to lose weight faster.

There are times when I cannot engage in my regular or preferred exercise, but is not procrastinating and avoiding exercise. I simply substitute another form of exercise for that period of time.

For example, I was recently aboard the beautiful cruise ship *Celebrity's Infinity* for two weeks. Most of the equipment in the gym was a little different for me, but I did engage in a great stretching program each morning that I did not leave early for an excursion. In Las Vegas I rose early ahead of the heat to get a walk and in Escondido repeated the same behavior. If in a hotel room for a couple of days, a large bath towel makes a great exercise mat.

Also aboard the cruise ship *Infinity*, I decided to do a body composition analysis (BCA). The result was pleasing. "You have a lot of bone and muscle tissue," I was told. Of course I was as pleased as having pie, even though there were more pounds to lose. So, I will continue to keep moving and watching what I eat. Surely the obesity problem will return, along with the diabetes threat or even a stroke or heart attack. So, I accept the challenge of being physically fit.

My grandnephew Corey came for a visit and was on the floor playing games. When I decided to join him, his grandfather, my brother Lynell, said, "Okay, when you get down there (on the floor), you may not be able to get up." Well, I got up when ready and with little effort, and was functionally fit, flexible, coordinated and with good balance. Again, I took pride in being fit.

At Baylor University a study was done by John Foreyt on exercise, nutrition and three approaches to weight loss. The study group included 127 men and women. Volunteers in Group one were put on a low-calorie diet. Group two exercised and took brisk walks three times a week. Group three was on a low-calorie diet and exercised three times a week. At the end of the first year, group one lost an average of 15 pounds. Group two lost an average of six pounds. Group three lost an average of 20 pounds after the second year, group one volunteers were heavier than when they started. Participants in group two regained all but five pounds of the weight lost. Only members of Group three held steady. Nutrition and exercise emerged as the best routine.

I do not like diets. No one is born to like diets, which is why they fail. A new approach is needed. Physical activity helps to maintain weight loss. Exercise is an important part of the answer, if you hate counting calories.

I conclude with an incident that makes all my exercising worthwhile. As I was leaving my car one beautiful, sunshiny morning headed for Sprouts Market in a white YMCA T-shirt and denims and no special hair-do, someone yelled out to me, "Diva!" Coming towards me was an unknown pretty young woman, probably in her mid-to-late-twenties.

"Who, me?" She was surprised by the look on my face. "Yes."

"I'm just an old woman,"

"No, honey, you're a diva!"

I graciously thanked her for the compliment. I put some pep in my steps, feeling as proud as any peacock. Wouldn't you?

CHAPTER 5

Sometimes Emotions
Get In the Way

*One of the greatest weight loss challenges is fighting
emotional eating – impulsive, unhealthy snacking triggered
by stress, boredom, depression, and other factors.*

- Bob Greene, fitness expert,
The Best Life Diet

TIME AND TIME AGAIN I have been "on a roll" with my weight loss and
exercise program, when something happened to disturb me or cause
emotional upset. The incident affected concentration on my goal.
Sometimes I took weeks or months to again reach that same level of
motivation. And, of course, it also provided a good excuse for allowing
my weight-loss efforts to be sabotaged.

Learning to identify what triggers emotional eating, cravings, and
backsliding is important. Not having problem foods available during
these times is a smart move and makes getting back on track easier
with fewer pounds to take off again.

My emotional mindset had a lot to do with my weight management
success. A good attitude must be supported by appropriate actions.
However, if preoccupied with other things, my actions were not always
in my best interests for conquering weight loss and achieving
maintenance. My hands were too busy feeding my face, usually with
wrong kind of food or too much of it.

In Bob Greene's book, *Get With the Program! Guide to Good Eating*, he advises that you should not let obligations to others interfere with obligations to yourself. Think of your health and well-being as sacred.

To change a stalled improvement effort and positive lifestyle changes, consider the following special interests: keep an exercise journal; rejuvenate a fitness program; revive a friendship; make new friends; join a social group...do something! Be action-oriented.

Do not expect instant change, but over the course of a year, you will experience positive substantial change if you can do one thing daily and consistently. Do three things consistently over a year, and you will have taken yourself out of a rut and probably will not recognize your former life. The changes may not be obvious on a day-to-day basis, but over the course of a year, the emotional eating will have vanished. Isn't that a great thought?

Notes

CHAPTER 5

Sometimes Medications Can Cause the Problem

"Mom, get off the Prednisone!"

- Brannon L. Woods, DVM

I WAS AT MY HEAVIEST WEIGHT after a prolonged use of prescribed Prednisone, a steroid used for allergic reactions and inflammation. Simply put, "it helps the body to function normally under abnormal conditions." My doctor warned me: "It'll put weight on you. Watch what you eat."

In addition to the weight gain, that medication can cause damage to the kidneys. The medication and the weight gain concerned my son, Brannon. So I took his advice, as he was very knowledgeable about pharmacology (like the Grady nurses in the next chapter). My son was a veterinarian.

As a nurse, familiar with the "tapering off" method safely took myself off Prednisone and told my doctor. *But I do not advise anyone to do what I did* because I know the process of "tapering-off" required to do it safely, myself having taught pharmacology for years. Be sure to check with your doctor, if you have any concerns.

Get Off the Prednisone!

Here I was at 265 pounds and still on the Prednisone. Having stayed on the drug at that point, I am not sure how much overweight would have overcome me.

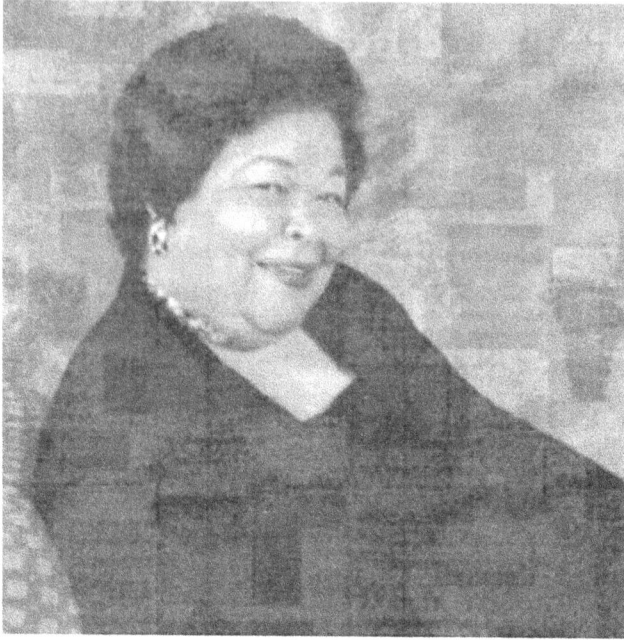

Mattie's Story

On a recent trip to Atlanta for my nursing class' 50th anniversary, the group had decided to have dinner together at a popular restaurant. About 27 of us were in town at that time.

"Mattie's going to be late," someone said.

We proceeded with dinner, laughing and teasing each other as usual. Then, this woman walked in and started talking to us.

"Who in the world's that?" I recall asking someone.

"That's Mattie Bryant," she said.

"Well, I wouldn't have recognized her in a million years."

Short and petite, Mattie's facial features were completely distorted. She was obese. When I approached her later, she said, "I was on Prednisone for ten years. I have Lupus and need to lose some weight."

Chances are weight loss will be more difficult for her, as Prednisone's residual remains in the body for some time.

While discussing the topic of Mattie's problem, another Grady colleague reported the recent death of a person on prolonged Prednisone use. Sad.

Lessons from Oprah

This discussion reminds me of one day seeing Oprah on her show, after I had taken a break from watching the program. She wore a full skirt, and her broad hips surprised me. I said to my friend, "Oprah's behind's as big as mine!" I was shocked by how much weight she had gained.

As health-and-fitness-conscious as Oprah is, I just knew she had to have a problem. Sure enough, I learned later that she was also having thyroid issues.

However, in a recent open letter to Oprah in *The Los Angeles Times,* James Fell (a certified strength and conditioning specialist from Calgary, Canada) told her that she had received poor advice about her thyroid problem as well as the need to exercise. He reminded her that she is "living proof" that a sustained motivation to exercise and eat right is necessary to maintain a desired weight. He suggested that she learn to "love exercise," rather than hate it, as she's admitted in the past. And he warned that falling in love with exercise is a gradual process. I agree.

Related Drug Categories

One day I stopped by my local pharmacy and asked about the categories of drugs that tend to cause weight gain. I was told that some antidepressants, anticonvulsants and sedatives have been associated with this problem.

The pharmacy tech added, "A lady just left who said she gained a hundred pounds while on an antidepressant."

"Which one?" I asked.

"I don't know, but the doctor changed it," the tech said.

As a former pharmacology instructor in nursing, I recognize that it is not possible to identify every drug or medication that tends to cause weight gain. There are literally thousands of drugs with side effects, interactions, various reactions, both with other drugs and the individual. Prednisone is an effective and popular drug whose weight-gaining side effects are known. Good monitoring is what is necessary.

Notes

_____

_____

_____

_____

_____

_____

_____

_____

_____

_____

_____

_____

_____

_____

_____

CHAPTER 7

Grady Nurses As
Priceless Diabetes Experts

*"From the very start of a career as an RN,
a nurse is not only a clinician,
but also a leader, teacher and scientist."*

- Jan Boller, PhD, RN

ABOUT EIGHTEEN MONTHS AFTER MY TRIP to Chicago to visit my brother, my journey took me to Birmingham, Alabama. I was going to attend a week-long conference with my nursing colleagues from Grady Memorial Hospital School of Nursing. Although the conference was held in Birmingham, the school of nursing was in Atlanta, a short distance away. I felt no stress, no fuss, and no bother. All vibes were good and positive, as my colleagues were generally "down-to-earth" people. My one concern was how well the group had maintained good health and normal weight.

My Training at Grady

On the way to the conference my thoughts drifted back several decades to 1958. For me, it was both the best and worst of times. It was the best of times, because it was an opportunity to further my education as a professional nurse. Not only was my class going to be the first one to be trained in the beautiful new Grady Hospital, but also we would be freshmen at Spelman College. I felt proud to be leaving Des Moines, Iowa to attend school in Atlanta. Old Dr. Hunter had told me that my ACT scores were among the highest in the group.

It was also the worst of times for me, because I had no idea how I was going to sustain myself financially for the next three years. It was bad enough missing the previous year, because of not having minimal tuition. Now, I didn't have a source of income for basic personal items, but went to school, anyway. My brother provided the financial support needed for the three years.

I was aware that Grady was segregated. The country was in the middle of social strife. However, it turned out to be a smaller problem than anticipated. All of us nursing students, blacks and whites, shared like facilities, equipment and space. In hindsight I now realize how much my Grady experience prepared me for the professional and social challenges of the next few decades.

Grady was then (and still is) a large urban hospital for the indigent. It is located less than a mile from the Centers for Disease Control and Prevention. Grady Hospital is a place where one never experiences boredom, especially on weekends. The Emergency Rooms were always filled with victims of trauma, heart attacks, strokes, asthmatic attacks or diabetic crisis. Gunshot wounds and stabbings only added to the problems. Hospital admissions always increased on weekends.

Nursing students at Grady were exposed to a multitude of challenging situations. By the time we were juniors and seniors, we were competent enough to assume charge responsibility for entire medical or surgical units or other nursing students. But we were bright and eager to help in any way we could. Though it was hard work, we were grateful for the opportunity to help others and learn.

Our patient population included a significant number of diabetic patients. We learned early about diabetic diets and "replacements" in our nutrition class and during rotations in the Diet Kitchen. We prepared thousands of diabetic diets with the required amounts of fats, carbohydrates and protein. The food was measured in grams for each 1000-cal, 1800-cal or 2000-cal diet. It was important that the patient maintained the diet ordered to counteract the amount of insulin taken before that meal; otherwise, the patient could have an untoward insulin reaction and somebody's head would roll. We knew to calculate what was consumed and to make a replacement for the portion not consumed.

The insulin administered before the patient ate was based on a sliding scale to determine how much sugar was being excreted into the urine before each meal. Depending on a color-coded dipstick reading of a 1+, 2+, 3+, or 4+ regular insulin was given according to this sliding scale. As well, a long-acting insulin was usually given in the morning.

At the time we graduated from Grady in the '60s, the standard diabetic treatment was mainly diet and insulin, and also how to take care of a "stump", if the person had an amputation. Seldom was there a diabetic crisis or problem. But the important bottom line here was that emphasis was on *treatment only*. Teaching the patient about the complications of diabetes and prevention was virtually non-existent. We didn't have the knowledge and information that we have today. The average diabetic patient today has better self-testing equipment than we used in the hospital at that time. Diabetics now are generally more knowledgeable about the disease, diet and exercise. Unfortunately, today there are millions of people who do not know they are diabetic or pre-diabetic.

Fast-Forward to the Conference

Getting back to the conference with my fellow Grady fellow-nurses, I was surprised to see that few of us were visibly overweight. My observation regarding our weight was not the same several years ago; I was plump at that time, as were others.

I shared my curiosity about the health and weight of our group of nurses with another Grady graduate, Clara Love, the conference chairperson. When she asked me about my current interests, I mentioned the Type II diabetes manuscript. She was quite encouraging. "It's a great challenge," she said. "It's something that's needed.

"You can do it."

Some 30 years later I was now hearing almost the exact same words I had heard earlier from Clara Love, who was also the supervisor for my first teaching assignment in the Los Angeles School District. I had a Regional Occupation Program (ROP) class teaching basic nursing skills to high school students at Hamilton High School. That teaching assignment turned out to be a nightmare, to say the least. At mid-semester three instructors had left their positions. The students had attitude problems, really serious attitude problems - not the kind with which you want to work in an acute hospital setting or the classroom.

Still, I was determined to give the teaching my best effort. When Mrs. Love took me to the school, she gave some lofty instructions to the principal about supporting me. Then she said, "Remember, you're a Grady graduate! You can do anything!"

I completed the school year, but it was a rough ride!

At the Grady conference Mrs. Love made similar observations about the nurses' group that I had, agreeing that most appeared to be a healthy weight. Near the end of the conference I was encouraged to do an impromptu survey. We were curious as to how the group felt about losing and regaining weight, which was easier or harder and what they considered the biggest obstacles to maintaining normal weight.

Sixty-one percent of the respondents said that it was harder to lose weight while thirty-nine percent said it was harder to maintain normal weight; and two wrote that both were a struggle. The biggest obstacles to losing weight were getting started, lack of time for exercise, lack of willpower, poor portion control, fast foods, eating out, social activities involving food and eating, as well as habits, boredom, and a lack of commitment. Try to identify your own obstacles from the following list.

Grady nurses made other pertinent comments about diabetes, disease, overweight and obesity which included:

- Some contributing factors are not caused by those involved (e.g., genetics, heredity and environment).

- The body mass index (BMI) does not differentiate between muscle tissue and fat tissue, or bone density. Therefore it should only be used as an indicator of being overweight.
- Overweight problems affect all organs of the body, leading to an unhealthy lifestyle.
- Overweight people need a change in lifestyle or alternative behavior.
- Fast-food restaurants contribute to the overweight problem, as do driving everywhere (instead of walking) and increased sedentary activities. In my field of psychiatry I found that medications increased weight.
- "Eat only when hungry" should be a constant rule.
- Some of the main problems in losing weight are learning to stop eating when you feel full and learning to drink more water.
- Servings are too large, exercise is too little, too much eating out and too little personal restraint.
- Flabby skin makes it hard to shop for clothes and having to continually get larger sizes.
- What we eat controls all systems of life.

The group concluded with comments about getting a copy of my book to the new Surgeon General and requesting that she use her influence to have food manufacturers decrease salt/sodium content in canned goods; decrease saturated fats; and use as little sugar as possible in sweets.

Although they were aware of the problems with and causes of diabetes, it was surprising to me that no one seemed to have remembered that when we were in training, *the emphasis was only on treatment, not prevention.* The patient had the disease, and that was that. Teaching such things as weight loss, exercise and good nutrition to prevent other family members from coming to the same fate was not done well. Most of our patient population did not know how to research diabetes on their own, as some patients do today. On the other hand, much of the information we have today was not in the past literature; otherwise, we, too, would have been better informed.

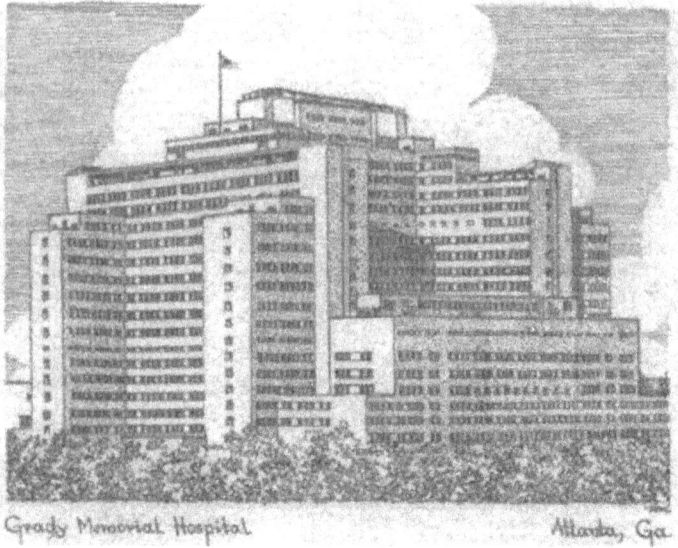

"Atlanta Can't Live Without Grady"
Grady Memorial Hospital
Atlanta, Georgia

Notes

_____

_____

_____

_____

_____

_____

_____

_____

_____

_____

_____

_____

_____

_____

CHAPTER 8

Inspiring Secret Success Strategies from Vegas and Other Places

"There are so many fad diets. If you want to change your life, you have to have good eating and exercise habits."

- Tyra Banks, Host,
America's Next Top Model

DISEASE REQUIRES A DIET, SPECIAL FOOD and a prescription, but a healthy lifestyle does not. I made a recent trip to Las Vegas, Nevada in search of ideas from others who have conquered the challenge of weight control with no special diet. I chose Las Vegas for a cross-section of information from all Americans and others, as well.

While much of this book deals with weight loss, I believe that learning to manage a normal healthy body weight is also important and is certainly a part of the premise on which a healthy lifestyle rests.

Observing Those Around Me

When boarding the plane in Los Angeles, I was thinking of the task of interviewing that awaited me in Las Vegas. I began making observations of the passengers on the plane. To my surprise, not one of them was visibly overweight. I found that discovery interesting. I asked myself, "Are we getting the weight-loss message?"

As I left the plane and headed for baggage claim, I received a reality check, which dashed my idea about Las Vegas visitors and residents being of normal weight. The good feeling vanished, as three loud, wide-bodied ladies took the escalator downstairs to the baggage claim area. The women told me that they were headed for the Riviera Hotel.

After I arrived at the resort to begin the interviews, two plump ladies ahead of me stood on the sidewalk. I immediately looked to my left and there, parked on a bench, were two obese women waiting for the shuttle for the casinos. One was puffing away on a cigarette, and I really had to restrain myself from saying something to her. I have two younger sisters, both of whom were smokers; they are currently being treated for cancer of the esophagus and emphysema. So I felt bad for the woman with the cigarette.

"Secret Success Strategies" from the Interviews

At any rate, I set out to interview those who appeared to be physically fit or who seemed to be of average weight and mobile. I wanted to learn their secrets. Some of their answers surprised me; others I had heard before. Either way, I believe you will find the information useful.

This particular strategy is new to me for weight control:

A Good Body Metabolism

"I was blessed with a good body metabolism, but I still try to eat right and exercise. I ride my bike to work."

- Liz, Las Vegas, 25.

Hunger Guides Eating

"I eat when I'm really hungry. I plan a nice meal, not just anything. Then I eat slowly, very slowly."

- Annabel, Sydney, Australia, 32

Fix the Brain First

"Fix the brain before you fix the body. Remember never to say 'diet' because the brain rejects the notion of diet and fights against it. Use portion control, or if you need to reduce, eat half of what you'd ordinarily eat - so you don't feel deprived."

- Joetta & Barbara, Los Angeles, 35 & 38

Control the Appetite

"I control my weight by controlling my appetite. I take one teaspoon of apple cider vinegar in a glass of warm water every morning. I don't experience hunger pangs during the day, so can eat sensibly."

- Carolyn Stamford, CT, 41

Diet and Exercise

"It's simply a matter of working out and watching what I eat."

- Chris, Eugene, Oregon, 25

The feedback during the survey provided for an interesting and successful project. In hindsight, though, I would conduct it differently by asking the participants to approach me or provide them with a written questionnaire. I believe the information would have been more in-depth.

Heading Back to LA

When it was time to return to Los Angeles, the plane was not full so an Asian woman changed her seat to sit beside me. She talked the whole hour, after learning my reasons for the interviews. Her name is Mae. She was 63 years of age and born in the People's Republic of China. She's never had a weight problem. It seems as though healthy eating has been a life-long endeavor.

I could relate to some of her childhood experiences. She spoke of having lots of fresh vegetables, while growing up, but not much meat. She ate fresh tomatoes from the vines with sugar, while I ate them with salt and pepper while on the farm in Mississippi. She ate watermelon, and so did I. Most or nearly all of our activities were done on our feet, walking.

Mae looked very healthy. She mentioned her diet and exercises. She chose brisk walking to other forms of exercise, such as yoga. Mae ate lots of vegetables and little meat.

Mae stated that she had made her physical well-being her top priority. Meanwhile, her husband was recovering from a stroke from stress at work.

Overall, Mae seemed happy. She mentioned that she was en route to Taiwan for her nephew's wedding.

Notes

_____

_____

_____

_____

_____

_____

_____

_____

_____

_____

_____

_____

_____

_____

CHAPTER 8

Our Reality
Reflected in Statistics

"Start treating as soon as the diagnosis is made.

- William C. Duckworth, MD
Veteran Affairs Diabetes Study

AN ASTOUNDING PREDICTION WAS MADE in a recent show, of January 6, 2011, *The Doctors:* "By the year 2030, eighty percent of the population will be obese" [if current trends continue]. This obesity pandemic will only increase the number of Type II diabetics and further impact the health-care system in a negative way.

Because Dr. Susan Davis is an efficient and proactive physician, she was able to alert me to my "pre-diabetes." My body did not suffer from the symptoms of diabetes, as happens to many who do not get an early diagnosis. Hopefully, other primary-care professionals will follow Dr. Davis' lead.

A Look at the Numbers

According to a recent Harris Poll Americans see obesity as a health threat on the same level as smoking. Eighty percent of Americans say obesity is "very harmful," compared to seventy-nine percent who say smoking is "very harmful."

Research shows that obesity can shorten one's life by five to ten years. According to a Rand Corporation study obesity is linked to more medical conditions than problem drinking and smoking. Obesity is costly to society.

Equally relative to obesity in general is the rise in the number of obese Americans. The fastest-growing group is comprised of people who are at least 100 pounds overweight. The number of obese children has also increased, along with an increase in the number of juvenile diabetics. The same physiological dynamics are probably at work - a lack of exercise, fast foods and sitting in front of TV's, computers and playing video games.

The number of disabled people is also expected to rise, as those with morbid obesity sustain weight-related muscular-skeletal problems and diabetes. If obesity trends progress at their current rate, up to one-fifth of healthcare expenditures could go toward treating the effects of obesity, causing nursing homes' expenses to grow 10 to 25 percent, thus taxing the Medicare and Medicaid systems.

America has a huge obesity problem. The unhealthy ratio is 1:3, and I was one of them at one time. More than 16 million people in the United States suffer from diabetes. Approximately 90 percent of all diabetics are Type II, and another 80 million are prediabetic.

Understanding Metabolic Syndrome

Diabetes often brings health problems, commonly called "metabolic syndrome." Persons have metabolic syndrome if they have at least three of the following conditions:

- You are overweight or obese and carry the weight around your middle. For men, this means a waist that measures greater than 40 inches around. For women, it means a waist measuring greater than 35 inches around.
- You have higher than normal blood pressure (130/85 mm Hg or greater).
- You have a higher than normal amount of sugar in your blood (A fasting blood sugar of 110 mg/dl or greater).
- You have a higher than normal amount of fat in your blood

(A triglyceride level of 150 mg/dl or greater).

- You have a lower than normal high-intensity lipoprotein (HDL) cholesterol level. HDL cholesterol is the good cholesterol. For men, this means an HDL level less than 40 mg/dl. For women, this means an HDL level less than 50 mg/dl.

The more of these risk factors you have, the higher your risk of heart disease.

A number of factors can act together to cause the metabolic syndrome. A person who takes in too many calories and too much saturated fat and does not get enough physical activity may develop metabolic syndrome. Other causes include insulin resistance and a family history of the risk factors for metabolic syndrome.

More Sobering Statistics

The Center for Disease Control and Prevention reported that no state met the Healthy People 2010 obesity target of 15 percent and the self-reported overall prevalence of obesity among US adults has increased 1.1 percentage points.

Wide sections of the Southeast, Appalachia and other tribal lands in the West and the Northern Plains have the nation's highest obesity and diabetes rates. In many counties in those regions rates of diagnosed diabetes exceeded ten percent and obesity is more than 30 percent (CDC, 2007).

Blacks had 51 percent higher prevalence of obesity, and Hispanics 21 percent, compared to whites (CDC, 2010).

In a segment aired on *The Doctors* in January, 2011, the number of people who go undiagnosed with diabetes each year was estimated at 80 million. During the past year, I have seen four new family members diagnosed with diabetes. All four had serious cases of the disease. However, none of the four knew they had diabetes. Medical insurance was not a problem, only a lack of awareness.

While genetics played a role in diabetes, obesity also was prevalent.

Therefore, we need more doctors who are proactive, like Dr. Davis, providing a better way to inform individuals at risk due to genetics and encouraging those overweight and obese to get tested.

Unfortunately, diabetics with high cholesterol also face the risk of heart attacks and cardiovascular disease. Controlling blood-sugar levels, lowering cholesterol and controlling high blood pressure reduces the risk of kidney and eye disease and other complications such as gangrene in the lower extremities, leading to amputation. Researchers found Type II diabetics have 65 to 75 percent chance of developing cardiovascular disease.

While Dr. William Duckworth (see quote at beginning of Chapter 9) recommends treating Type II diabetes early, the problem is identifying diabetics before a heart attack or stroke happen possibly seriously damaging the person's health. Duckworth believes "blood pressure and lipid control," along with an "improved diet and exercise and treatment with aspirin" will save lives.

I have no valid reason to disagree, and this is precisely the path that Dr. Davis and I have taken in my case.

Notes

_____

_____

_____

_____

_____

_____

_____

_____

_____

_____

_____

_____

_____

_____

CHAPTER 10

Are You Ready?
"When someone makes an appointment to see
me, I assume they're ready. But then I see other
people who are told by their physician to see me.
When I ask why they're here, they say, 'I don't know.
My Dr. sent me.' And I know they're not ready.

- Dr. Jorge Vasquez,
Director of Medical Nutrition,
Allegheny Center for Digestive Health, Pittsburgh

THE SUCCESS THAT PEOPLE ACHIEVE with nutritional weight-management depends on how ready they are. This statement is true of counseling, taking a new job, marriage and most tasks. It's the readiness factor that counts. I started many times when I was not ready.

What the Experts Say

Comments of experts in the area of behavioral health are helpful in understanding our motivation, commitment and satisfaction with nutritional endeavors.

Jeannine Stein, Los Angeles Times health writer says, "Weight loss requires an overhaul of diet (nutrition consumed), exercise and essentially your entire life. But putting off these changes is a national pastime. Eating right and exercising is better done next week because today just isn't the right time."

To lose weight, say experts in nutrition and weight loss, you must be r-e-a-d-y to make changes, even small ones. Nutrition researchers even came up with a Weight Loss Readiness Test, a questionnaire sometimes used by health professionals and individuals to determine levels of motivation and commitment and to examine connections with food and exercise.

But what does "being ready" really mean and how do you know when you're there? These specialists discuss the readiness factor:

- **Martin Binks,** Director of Behavioral Health and Research at the Duke Diet and Fitness Center in Durham, North Carolina and co-author of The Duke Diet, says: "I would rephrase that as 'What would I be willing to change? Among these things, where do I start?' The diet mentality is that you suddenly go from 100 to zero tomorrow, the on/off mentality. Identifying what a person's barriers are to losing weight, he adds, is key: "For one person, it might be work commitments; for another, emotional upheavals. But what could you start to change now?"

- **Jorge Vasquez, MD** (see his quote at the beginning of Chapter 10) further states that "there should be deeper motivations than looking good for a reunion or a wedding." That's a perceptive statement! He goes on to say: "Better ones are that you want to feel better, be healthier, and not take insulin anymore."

- **Kathleen Zelman,** an Atlanta-based registered dietitian, and the Director of Nutrition for WebMD, says: "The precise moment of readiness is different for everyone. For people who have been successful at losing weight, something happens in their lives that triggers an 'a-ha' moment. It could be having the doctor tell them that if they don't lose weight, they're going to die. I don't know if you say, 'I'm ready,' but you feel like you can't go on like this." She adds that being 100 percent prepared isn't always a prerequisite.

"Even if you're not ready, see if you can make some changes that are doable. If you're a couch potato, go for a walk...do something that you like for fifteen minutes. Once you see some benefits - you're sleeping better, you have more energy– then maybe that will give you a spark, and hopefully that will lead you to say, 'Now I'm ready to be more serious, and I'll step it up.'"

- **Dr. David Heber,** Director of UCLA's Center for Human Nutrition, agrees that "The stimulus is different for different people." He recognizes that this statement could mean a negative health diagnosis from a doctor for one person or an anticipated social event for another. In any case, having a plan and a reasonable weight-loss goal is paramount for success, Hebner advises.

I was ready at the time, when Dr. Davis told me I was "prediabetic", as soon as I recovered from an initial state of shock and disbelief!

CHAPTER 11

Just Do It for Success!

"...the ones who understand that this is a process [know] that what they are doing is changing their relationship with food."

- Dr. Howard M. Shapiro Author,
Picture Perfect Weight Loss

ACCORDING TO HOWARD M. SHAPIRO, MD (and I agree), "Diets are boring. Food is not." The first day in the process will probably be your hardest, if you lack willpower, hunger pangs may set in before your next feeding, so, be tolerant. As the stomach adjusts to having less food, it will shrink, and the urge to eat will diminish over time. Plan the first day well and the following days will become easier as the week progresses. Then take pride in getting through one week.

More Supportive Tips

Keep in mind the old maxim: If you do something for twenty-one days, it becomes a habit. Now, I ask you, what more important habit could you have than adopting a lifelong nutrition plan to gain and maintain normal weight? The plan is safe, healthy and interesting. We tire of diets, but never tire of food. We can always change our choices. Change can be your first step on a lifelong journey.

On a prescribed diet we become bored and "fall off the wagon." A full variety of choices makes planning more interesting. Remember, if you tend to eat all day, selecting five or six small meals may be preferable to three large meals.

Initially, you will need, as I did, to get yourself oriented to just how much a cup, or a portion of a cup, is. Measuring cups and spoons help. A small food scale for meat portions comes in handy, while you're making the adjustment.

The two most important actions you can take are jotting down what you eat each day and weighing yourself. If you gain weight, go back and look at what you ate the day before. Chances are you had a larger meal(s) or extra snacks. Sometimes when shopping, I get a bit too interested in the samples. The scales remind me the next day of the danger of such sampling.

Divide large snack portions into single-portion sizes. Don't buy the goodies or treats you find irresistible. Tell your friends that you're making a lifestyle change, which you're leaving behind "weight-loss diets," because they do not work. Explain that we become bored with these kinds of diets and gain back the weight lost. Ask for your friends' support as well as that of your family: To prevent diabetes, their support is extremely important.

Prolonged deprivation may lead to binging. Experts say that it's permissible to give yourselves a treat, as long as we include it in our daily or weekly plan. Treats may include low-fat ice cream, 1/4 cup of peanuts in the shell, or three pieces of chocolate.

Exercise Is Essential

Included in any healthy weight-loss plan is some form of exercise. Professionals encourage walking. However, dancing, swimming, and gym workouts are also effective. About 10,000 steps per day are adequate, if you choose walking. A pedometer can be useful to count your steps. Standing is better than sitting, but walking is better than standing.

Notes

_____

_____

_____

_____

_____

_____

_____

_____

_____

_____

_____

_____

_____

_____

_____

CHAPTER 12

My Changes and Remaining Challenge

"The key is to make lifestyle changes you can stick with long-term (like walking)."

- Malissa J. Wood, MD
Women's Heart Health Program,
Massachusetts General Hospital

THE CHALLENGE TO MAKE LIFESTYLE CHANGES requires planning and commitment. Of the two main areas of planning, one is a change in eating patterns and the amount and the second is a change in activity or exercise. Willpower is needed for these two changes, and I am committed to both.

To Look at Eating

A change in eating patterns means that you must examine not only what you eat but when and how much. For example, a regular breakfast of bacon, eggs, grits, sausage or ham, pancakes and hash browns pales beside a breakfast of whole-wheat cereal, light soymilk and fresh fruit or a similar breakfast, such as non-fat cottage cheese, fruit and whole-wheat toast, or oatmeal and berries. You get to select your choice.

Similarly, planning lunch to avoid rich fast foods, such as fries and burgers, and rich sweet treats offers another interesting challenge.

Salads, broiled meat, fish or tofu and baked chips are better choices. The sugary drinks do not help, either.

You also should plan well for dinner. I know that, for me, sometimes coming home from work tired and hungry encourages unhealthy eating. Pre-planning is very important to what I am going to have. Steak, white rice, macaroni and cheese, potato salad and all the white rolls and butter I can eat are not ideal dinner selections I could plan. On the other hand, a broiled chicken breast, three asparagus stalks and brown rice are ideal. Just think about how much fun it can be planning healthy, wholesome meals that you like and find interesting and fulfilling. Just plan ahead to avoid wrong choices.

Between breakfast, lunch, dinner and bedtime, you also need to plan for snacks. A snack should not be equivalent to a meal. On the market now are such things as healthy snack granola bars of 100 calories and mini-rice cakes of 90 calories. Apples make great snacks or a handful of raisins or another fruit. Some enjoy celery sticks with low-fat peanut butter or cottage cheese. Be curious and creative to select snacks you like which are non-fattening.

Remember, if you have a food weakness, as I did with peanuts, don't buy them and bring the problem food into your home. Also, get rid of all other problem foods. Shop for healthy, non-fattening foods, vegetables and fruits. Study the My Plate Guide from Chapter 3 for the recommended number of servings per day. The serving-size chart of meat, fish, eggs, vegetables and fruits, and rice will help control portion size. Both servings per day and serving size selected from the My Plate Guide and serving-size chart are very helpful in weight control and weight loss.

Another important factor to remember is to use a food diary or a food guide. Write what you had for breakfast, snack, lunch, snack, dinner, and snack. Note whether you were able to stick to the guidelines for number of servings and serving size; if not, why were you unable to do so? Then, think through what caused you to overeat. What will you do differently the next day? Take the appropriate steps.

What about Exercise?

A change in activity is also necessary. Exercise in some form is a must. To lose weight faster, increase the amount of exercise. Decide what form of exercise you like and commit to doing it.

Refining Your Approach

It's important to examine your attitude towards being overweight, food and exercise. The choice is yours to make a change. You may choose to take action or continue habits the way they are, depending on your condition. Learn as much as you can about food and nutrition and the relationship of exercise. Make healthy eating and exercise habits. Take a multivitamin, and drink six to eight glasses of water per day.

See how you can best divide your meals and snacks. I prefer three small meals and three snacks. Some people prefer three regular meals. Others include three snacks. However, should you establish regular healthy eating habits and suddenly go on a binge, don't beat up on yourself and keep binging. Get back on the wagon as soon as you can. Effort becomes easier over time, because it is a habit.

If eating out is a problem for you, as it was for me, take the helpful hint both my personal physician and Pamela Lee gave to me. "Eat half of your meal and take the other half to go."

Remember, "diets" don't work! We get tired eating the same food or bored with the same food, then stop that diet. The weight returns and we select another diet. The process repeats itself along with the problems of being overweight. So, what is needed is a change in regular eating habits and exercise that will have a long-term effect on normal body weight.

Lastly, always discuss weight-loss problems with your health-care professional before you begin a program. One half-pound per week or two pounds per month are usually recommended. An attempt to "quick-fix" the problem is considered unhealthy and risky.

A Word about Backsliding

Backsliding is common and expected, and we should not beat up on ourselves or feel guilty. We just get back to where we left off as soon as we can. Just think about the circumstances. The gain may be small or great, but the "yo-yo" effect is always a danger. I know because I have been there.

Try It...It Works!

No other diet action or procedure than self-management combined with exercise and the appropriate nutrition has given me a solution to my weight problem. I am aware of my sluggish metabolism, and therefore must seek a combination of foods, herbs and exercise that will boost my metabolism for further weight loss and weight maintenance. In other words, staying power is working just fine, and I continue on a path to a healthier, happier lifestyle. Please join me!

Notes

_____

_____

_____

_____

_____

_____

_____

_____

_____

_____

_____

_____

_____

Afterword

"Athlete!"

"What did you say?" I asked.

"I said you're an athlete," the phlebotomist told me as he put the tourniquet on my arm. "I can tell by the muscles."

Of course I felt like I was wearing a halo!

That was January 3, 2012. I was giving a blood specimen for Dr. Davis. The young technician told me he was pre-diabetic but, had found out in time to help prevent it. "I like cookies," he said.

"What's your A1C?" I asked him.

"It's 6.1."

"Okay, but you need to work a little harder." "Mine's 5.3."

Well, it was 5.3 until this latest reading. Now it had gone up to 5.4. I had a feeling it could have been higher than that at some point since the last reading. I was not surprised because I failed to follow my own advice.

You see, I insisted on cooking Thanksgiving dinner. I made all the things I liked, such as cornbread stuffing and yams and fresh creamed corn. One meal led to another and before I knew it, I had seven unwanted pounds to lose all over again.

My advice to you is this: Don't put yourself in a "vulnerable situation" as I did. A simple meal at Thanksgiving dinner would have been just fine. Having all the leftovers was like being at a continuous all-you-can-eat buffet.

Since then I have found that the lychee berry extract helps me to crave less food during late-afternoon and evenings. It appears to have the same effect on me that cinnamon has at breakfast. Dr. Oz regularly recommends one teaspoonful, but I prefer the capsule.

Planned weight loss for me has occurred over the last several years. It was not and should not be a quick-fix process. During this time I have acquired regular exercise habits and a better appreciation for disciplined healthy eating. It's been a great journey!

Sometimes, I feel like singing the old Negro spiritual:

"I know I've been changed,

Oh, I know I've been changed, I know I've been changed,

The angels in Heaven done signed my name."

Let me leave you with these three important points involving changes in your habits, food and physical activity: (1) Change should become a part of your lifestyle in terms of what you eat and your daily movements. (2) The changes need not be sudden or painful. My 60-pound weight loss has been gradual, yet effective. (3) Don't be hard on yourself, if you backslide.

Doctors and dietitians advise losing weight gradually, because you are then much more likely to achieve permanent weight loss. Challenge yourself for this goal. Remember, this is a journey, not a destination.

I know from personal experience that old and bad habits are hard to break. It's tough to change what you eat and the way you feel about food after years of habitual poor choices. So, if you one day revert to your old but high-calorie favorites, don't despair. Simply start where you left off, before you strayed. On days that I break my nutrition plan, I "fine" myself by dropping a quarter into the kitty.

There are no shortcuts to weight loss, either in food intake or exercise. Very few of us can eat whatever and whenever we like without paying; a price in pounds. A proper diet and physical movement are vital for healthy, physiological functioning. Challenge yourself to see what benefits you. It worked for me and will work for you.

The road to healthy living is open. TAKE IT!

APPENDICES

APPENDIX A

The Be Well Program

I'd never seen such a systematic, positive, strong finding.
The results were so astonishing that I didn't believe them.
I thought my colleagues were playing a joke on me.

- Lester Breslow, MD
Dean, UCLA's Fielding
School of Public Health

WHAT A POWERFUL AND AMAZING statement by Dr. Breslow! He was referring to the news he had gotten about the results of a study on the "Seven Habits of Healthy Living".

I believe his response would be similar to the results found in a current on-going program called Be Well, which is great for a healthy lifestyle. The purpose for sharing this information is to inspire others to develop such programs to maintain health, well-being and prevent disease. However, before moving on to "Be Well," a discussion about Dr. Lester Breslow seems to be in order. His influence on disease prevention was profound. He played an important pioneering role in making the transition from simply treating disease to a much wider effort to preventing disease.

As previously stated, the initial quote made reference to the results of a study by Dr. Breslow and his group did using the Seven Habits of Healthy Living. The team reported to Dr. Breslow that a 45-year-old person who had adhered to at least six of the seven habits had a life expectancy 11 years longer than peers who followed fewer than four of the habits. A 60 year-old who followed all seven of the habits was as healthy as a 30 year-old who followed two or less of the habits.

Dr. Breslow's Seven Habits of Healthy Living followed in the study were:

Regular breakfast;

Exercise;

Regular sleep;

Non-smoking;

Drinking in moderation or not at all;

Eating regular meals with no in between snacking;

Maintaining normal weight.

Healthy habits are important to disease prevention. The Be Well program is an excellent on-going nutrition and exercise program for those over 55 and has a health concern such as hypertension, overweight, high cholesterol, stiffness, etc. I am convinced about the merits of the program because having seen remarkable results occur in many of the participants. Several of those attending the program shared their experiences with me:

An inspiring and educational class that keeps bones moving that ordinarily wouldn't be moving.

- Marlene Denmore

The Be Well Program saved my life! From an obese, depressed, frightened "new" senior to a fit, happy, joy-filled "seasoned" senior. I emerged full of vigor and life. The brilliance of this program cannot be praised enough. I have the mindset of a 20 year-old. I was at the 1964 Olympics. Thank you, Be Well Program!!!

- Marilyn White

An excellent program. It is informative, encouraging and rejuvenating! Kudos to the Inglewood Senior Center.

- Jeanette Parish, Ed. D.

I have been in the "Be Well" class for five months. It has been a blessing to me. I learned how to eat healthy and combined it with exercise. I have been inspired to continue on this health maintenance road. I love every step I have taken and will keep on pushing forward.

I lost 11 pounds, several inches off my waist and my cholesterol has significantly decreased. My overall health has improved. Thank you, "Be Well"! I am a new woman because of you!

- Marie Wakefield

"Be Well" has helped me take better control of my health in terms of blood pressure, blood sugar and cholesterol. My doctor at Kaiser encouraged me to keep-up the good work. She now sees me every six months instead of every three months.

- Veda Neal

Since taking classes (the "Be Well" Program) at Darby Park my bad knees have become much better. They are not stiff as before.

- Bill Rifer

The Be Well Program is great for seniors. It teaches the importance of good nutrition as well as daily exercise. You learn the various food group exchanges and the amount of calories they contain. This helps you plan your meals accordingly. Those who need to lose weight can learn how it's done. I recommend this program to all seniors even those who do not need to lose weight.

- Dolores Chavous

I have lost approximately 15 pounds by utilizing what I learned in the nutrition part of the program! Thanks, Be Well!

- Lydia Jourdan

For several years I have been involved with the Be Well program. It is great! I have learned a lot.

I am diabetic and I am able to keep my diabetes under control. The nutrition part enables me to eat the correct food and proper amount. I can read food labels better, too. Exercise keeps me fit. I can stretch and avoid diabetic neuropathy.

- Patricia Templeton

The program is much more thorough and in-depth than this simple outline indicates; in other words, it is well-developed:

Topic/Presentation/Discussion

Introduction/Orientation
Functional Fitness Test
Role of Exercise
Personalized Exercise Plan
Personalized Food Management Plan
Changing How You Eat
Reading Nutrition Labels
Identifying Hidden Fat
Sodium Control with Dash Diet
Why Fad Diets Fail
Planning for Success
Developing a Support System
Healthy Low-calorie Snacks
Solo Cooking
Holiday Survival and Setbacks
Final Testing-Lab Tests
Celebration!

I have enjoyed being a participant/observer in the Be Well Program. I have learned new information and been reminded of some forgotten. Should you have the opportunity to participate, don't pass it up!

Note: The Be Well Program is funded by the L.A. County Department of Aging, the Kaiser Permanente Foundation, the City of Inglewood, California, and the Community Foundation. Contact their consultants for program information.

Appendix B

Warning Signs of Type II Diabetes

You may have no warning signs at all. Or you may have the following signs:

- Increased thirst
- Increased hunger
- Fatigue
- Increased urination, especially at night
- Weight loss
- Blurred vision
- Sores that do not heal
- Tingling or numb feet and hands

It is important to remember that there are millions of people who don't know they have diabetes. Get tested.

Source: *The Healthy Woman*
US Department of Health and Human Services
Office of Women's Health, 2010

APPENDIX C

Heart Attack Warning Signs

- Light-headedness
- Pain, discomfort, numbness in the arms, back, jaw, neck or between shoulders
- Pain, pressure, fullness or squeezing of the chest
- Cold sweating of the skin
- Difficulty breathing (shortness of breath)
- Upset stomach; urge to throw up
- May feel tired, have heartburn, a cough, fluttering of the heart or a loss of appetite.

IF YOU THINK YOU ARE HAVING A HEART ATTACK, WAIT NO MORE THAN FIVE MINUTES BEFORE CALLING 911. You must act quickly to prevent disability or death.

Source: *The Healthy Woman*
US Department of Health and Human Services Office of Women's Health, 2010

Appendix D

Stroke Risk Factors and Warning Signs

Stroke Risk Factors

- High blood pressure
- Heart disease, especially an irregular heartbeat known as Atrial Fibrillation (AF)
- Smoking
- Diabetes
- High cholesterol
- Obesity/poor diet
- Over age 50

Stroke Warning Signs

- Sudden numbness or weakness in face, arm or leg
- Sudden difficulty speaking
- Sudden severe dizziness, loss of balance or coordination
- Sudden dimness, loss of vision
- Sudden, intense headache
- Brief loss of consciousness

Source: *The Healthy Woman*
US Department of Health and Human Services
Office of Women's Health, 2010

APPENDIX E

My Obesity-buster Fitness Kit

- A set of measuring spoons: for accuracy
- A set of measuring cups for accuracy
- A food scale to weigh accurately, until able to eyeball a portion
- A pedometer to track the number of steps taken each day. Recommended goal is 10,000 steps. You are considered sedentary, if less than 4,000 steps are taken each day.
- A measuring tape to track inches lost
- A food diary to keep a record of what is eaten each day, how much, and when it was consumed. The diary is a valuable weight-loss tool.
- Comfortable clothes for exercising; dress appropriately for the weather.
- May use light hand-weights of about one or two pounds to start.
- Good athletic walking shoes

APPENDIX F

Pounds. Pounds, Pounds to Go!

*Weight loss alone will have a significant
impact on many aspects of overall health.*

- Julian Whitaker, MD

WHILE WEIGHT LOSS FOR ME HAS BEEN SLOW and gradual, according to Dr. Davis' advice, others have been successful with different strategies and choices. The key for all of us is to make lifestyle changes with which that we can live. I discourage the use of injections, pills, surgery and weight-loss centers; they provide a temporary fix for a long-term problem and can be dangerous.

One weight-loss success story is about a person who attends my church. She was determined to lose weight and keep it off. For the last several years she has run the Los Angeles Marathon. This year, she was the leader of her training group. I'm very proud of Cynthia. Here's what she did:

Ask a Friend

"Each week at church I noticed a friend who looked smaller as the weeks went by. I finally asked her what her secret was. She invited me to a meeting of Food Addicts, where I found the secret to losing and maintaining my weight: Eliminating sugar, flour and fried foods from my daily eating, as well as weighing and measuring my foods, along with training for marathons year-round, I have been able to maintain my weight loss."

- Cynthia Matthews, 59, Los Angeles, CA lost 43 pounds

During my interviews in Las Vegas a lady overheard me talking to someone else. She volunteered herself to provide information on weight loss:

Protein Shakes

"I tried everything. Then someone told me about protein shakes. Over a period of one year, I lost one hundred pounds without exercising. I kept it off until I injured my hip and became less active."
- Marie Van Pelt, 73, Las Vegas; lost 100 pounds

Doctors had advised my friend's husband to lose weight, and his wife was very supportive. During a six-month period he lost weight, using certain conscious eating techniques. Here is what they said:

Eat Slowly. Eat More Often, But Eat Less

"Don't eat in front of the TV. Chew. Chew. Chew. Pick foods that have some crunch, so you must chew more, such as cut-up veggies, apple slices, and popcorn or rice cakes. The reason we suggest this is that we believe it takes twenty to thirty minutes for your stomach to tell your brain that you're full.

"Eat more often, but eat less. This way, you have a steady amount of food to fuel your body and avoid indigestion, constipation and mood problems.

Albert has lost twenty-six pounds."
- Albert and Donna Jacard, Beverly Hills

One of my editors found that unwanted extra pounds had crept up during an emotional period. She chose a familiar food choice to jumpstart her weight-loss campaign.

Starvation

The Rev. Al Sharpton, 57, was asked how he lost so much weight. He responded this way:

"About eleven years ago I led a protest in Puerto Rico on the island of Vieques and we were able to successfully stop the U.S. Navy from bombing exercises. For the sit-in I was given 90 days in jail, so decided to go on a hunger strike for 40 days. I just had liquid, lost a lot of weight, and started feeling and looking better.

I ran for president in 2004 and my weight started going back up because of all the dinners and room service. I was around 240, 250. So I went on a self-imposed diet, where I ate salads, chicken and fish and drank coffee and tea. In the last year I cut that out, no coffee, and no chicken. I'm down to 160, 165 and I feel better."

- Irene Lacher Calendar Section
Los Angeles Times
February 19, 2012

Cabbage Soup to Start

"My weight gain was largely emotional. But at a certain point, I didn't want to add on any additional pounds. A friend had used the Cabbage Soup Diet, and so I tried it as a way to begin my weight- loss program. After a week on it, I had decreased my appetite. Then I went to 1400 calories a day, measuring all my foods and just generally making healthy choices. I've also heard that 1600 calories a day is a good goal for weight loss. I increased my exercise, too, aiming for thirty to forty-five minutes of walking a day - at least five days a week. Sometimes I'd go to the gym, and other days, I'd walk around the neighborhood. In addition, I did stretching, which helped keep my body limber. To deal with my emotions, I turned to journaling and breathe work. I also distracted myself with funny movies at night, to avoid the nighttime eating that so easily adds on the pounds — especially when carbs are involved! It was so exciting to reach my goal weight, and to fit into the smaller sized jeans that had been at the bottom of my dresser!"

- Robin Quinn, Los Angeles; lost 30 pounds

Cabbage soup is made with a medium head of cabbage, one green bell pepper, one large yellow onion, a bunch of celery and a 14-ounce can of diced tomatoes. Add enough low-sodium chicken broth or water to cover before boiling. A half-pound of lean ground turkey or chicken may be added after it has been browned, if desired.

APPENDIX G

Upper Body Flexibility Exercises
"Courtesy of Fit Linxx, Inc. 2011"

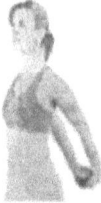

Anterior Deltoid, Chest and Bicep Stretch

Sit or stand with your hands clasped behind your back. With your shoulder blades squeezed together and your shoulders pressing down toward the floor, keep your chest up and slowly lift your arms up towards the sky as far as you comfortably can. You should feel the stretch across your upper chest, biceps and shoulders. Hold for 30 seconds. Do not bounce.

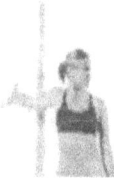

Chest Stretch

Stand facing a tree or wall. Extend an arm straight out to the wall at shoulder height with your palm against the wall and thumb up. Turn your body away from your extended arm. You should feel the stretch on the front side of your armpit and across the front of your chest. Hold for 30 seconds. Switch sides and repeat.

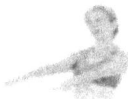

Hands

Clench both hands into fists. Hold for 10 seconds. Stretch your fingers as far apart as possible. Hold for 10 seconds.

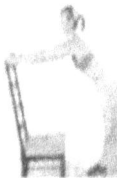

Lat Stretch for the Back

Stand straight with toes, hips, knees and shoulders facing forward. Place both hands shoulder-width apart on a fence or ledge and let your upper body drop down as you bend your knees slightly. Hold for 30 seconds. Do not bounce. Keep your knees bent when coming out of this stretch.

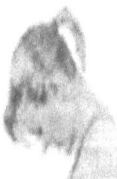

Neck - Chin to Chest Stretch

(All movements should be slow and easy. Do not roll your head around or ex- tend your head backward when looking up. This compresses spine.) Stand or sit straight. While looking straight ahead, slowly drop your chin to your chest. Hold for 10 seconds. Slowly return to starting position.

Upper Body Flexibility Exercises, continued

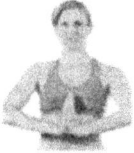

Wrist Extension

While seated or standing, bring both hands together at chest height with your palms together. Slowly press your hands together harder as you drop your hands from chest height down towards your navel. Hold for 30 seconds.

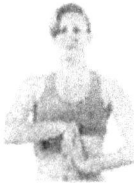

Wrist Flexion

While seated or standing, bring your right arm in towards your body, bent at the elbow. Your right hand should be just above your navel, knuckles up, palm facing the ground. Place your left hand over your right hand. Flex your wrist as far as you comfortably can by dropping your hand so your fingers point to the ground. Use the other hand to push slightly on the hand to increase the stretch. Hold for 30 seconds. Switch arms and repeat.

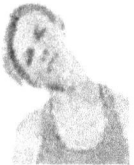

Neck - Ear to Shoulder Stretch

(All movements should be slow and easy. Do not roll your head around or extend your head backward when looking up. This compresses your spine.) Stand or sit straight. While looking straight ahead, let your head slowly fall to the left side, with your left ear toward your left shoulder. Do not force it. Hold for 10 seconds. Perform the same exercise on the right side. Hold for 10 seconds.

Overhead Stretch for Chest and Shoulders

Stand straight with arms overhead crossed at the wrists and palms together. Stretch your arms up and very slightly back as high as you comfortably can. Press your hands together firmly. Feel the stretch in your intercostal muscles, upper back, and interior shoulder. Hold the stretch for 30 seconds. Do not bounce.

Shoulder Stretch across the Chest

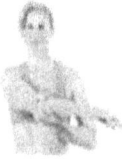

Place your right arm across your chest, keeping your arm straight and your shoulders down. Bring your left arm up from underneath, place it just above the elbow and actively but gently pull your right arm toward your body. You should feel the stretch across the top of your shoulder and upper arm. Hold for 30 seconds. Do not bounce. Switch sides and repeat.

Triceps' & Shoulder Stretch

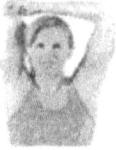

Stand straight with your arms overhead. Bend your left arm at the elbow. Reach down with your left hand and touch the base of your neck. Bend your right arm at the elbow and rest your right hand on your left elbow. Gently pull your left elbow back behind you. Hold for 30 seconds. Do not bounce. Switch arms and repeat.

Upper Back and Rotator Cuff Stretch

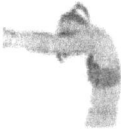

Raise your arms to shoulder height straight in front of you. Intertwine your fingers and turn your palms away from your body. Push your hands away from your body until you feel the stretch under and across your shoulder blades. Take a deep breath in and let your chin fall to your chest as you exhale. You should feel the stretch in your upper back. Hold for 30 seconds, breathing normally. Do not bounce.

APPENDIX H

Lower Body Flexibility Exercises
"Courtesy of Fit Linxx, Inc. 2011"

Seated Gluteus Stretch for Buttocks

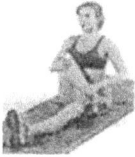

Sit on the floor or on an exercise mat, with your spine straight, shoulders back and both legs extended straight out ahead of you. Lift your right leg and cross it over your left, placing your heel flat on the ground. Place both hands on your right knee and gently pull your knee into your chest while maintaining the straight posture in your spine until you feel a stretch on the outside of your hip and into your buttock. Hold for 30 seconds. Do not bounce. Switch legs and repeat.

Single Leg Crossover Stretch for Lower Back and Glute

Lie flat on your back on the floor. Keep your entire back and your head flat on the floor. Bring one leg up towards your chest, bend your knee at 90 degrees and, while guiding with your opposite hand, let that leg fall across your body until your knee reaches the floor. Now, place gentle pressure on the outside of your knee using that same hand until you feel the stretch across your lower back and outside of your hip. Keep your feet and ankles relaxed. Make sure your shoulders are flat on the floor. If the angle between your shoulders and hips changes, it becomes difficult to create a proper stretch. Hold an easy stretch for 30 seconds on each side. Do not bounce.

Standing Hamstring Stretch

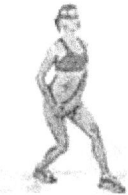

Stand straight with shoulders, hips, knees and toes forward. Take a big step forward with your left leg. Bend your right leg to about 90 degrees as you sit back with your weight on your right leg. Place both hands on top of your right, thigh for support. Keep a slight bend in the left leg while it is extended out in front of the body, with your left foot flat on the floor. As you sit back on your right leg with your chest and chin up, feel the stretch in the back of your left thigh. Hold for 30 seconds. Do not bounce. Switch legs and repeat.

Standing Hip Flexor Stretch for Groin

Standing straight up, step forward with your right foot. With hips, knees, and toes forward, raise your left heel off the floor. With the weight of your left leg on the ball of your left foot, push forward with your hips while keeping both feet on the floor. You should feel the stretch at the top of your left thigh, just under your hip bone. Hold for 30 seconds. Switch sides and repeat.

Standing Quadriceps Stretch

Stand straight with toes, hips, and shoulders facing forward. Lift your left foot off the ground, bending at the knee as if you are trying to kick your buttock with your heel. Stand straight; do not lean forward at your hips. Grab your ankle with your left hand and keep standing straight. You should feel the stretch in your left thigh. Hold for 30 seconds. Switch sides and repeat.

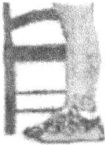

Ankle

Stand on one leg using a chair, wall, or bar for support. Raise the other leg about 45 degrees off the floor. Point the foot of the raised leg. Hold for 10 seconds. Now flex the foot and hold for 10 seconds. Repeat 5 times, then switch legs and repeat.

Butterfly Stretch for Inner Thigh

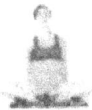

Sit on the floor or on an exercise mat. Put the soles of your feet together and hold onto your ankles. Sit straight up with your shoulders back and your chest and chin up. Lower your knees to the floor as far as you comfortably can until you feel a good stretch in your groin. Hold for 30 seconds. Do not bounce.

Calf Stretch

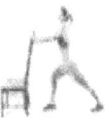

Stand a few steps away from a wall, tree or other solid support with your arms outstretched. Step forward with one leg, bend it at the knee and place your foot on the ground in front of you and your hands on the wall for support. The opposite leg remains straight behind you. Slowly lean forward, keeping your spine straight. Keep your shoulders, hips, knees and toes forward. Keep both feet flat on the ground. Hold an easy stretch for 30 seconds. Do not bounce. Switch legs and repeat.

Lower Body Flexibility Exercises, continued

Cat Stretch for Back

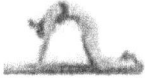

Start out on your hands and knees, which should be shoulder width apart. Flatten your back while relaxing your hips. Exhale as you curl your back so that it arches through the center of your spine (like a cat). Hold for 30 seconds. Relax back to your starting position.

Cobra Stretch for Lower Back

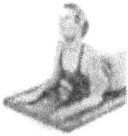

Lie on your stomach with your arms out ahead of you and legs straight. Start with your palms and your feet flat on the floor. Slowly arch up with your upper body as you walk your hands in towards your body. Keep your hips and toes on the floor. Press up on your hands as you reach with your chest towards the sky while pushing down through your hips into the ground. Keep your leg muscles relaxed throughout the entire motion. You should feel this stretch in your lower back and you may also feel a stretch in your abdominals depending on your flexibility. Hold for 30 seconds.

Knees to Chest Stretch for Lower Back

Lie flat on your back on the floor. Keep your entire back and your head flat on the floor. Slowly bring your knees up toward your chest, one at a time. Hold your legs behind the knees and gently pull towards your chest for an extra stretch. Be sure to keep your lower back flat against the floor. Hold an easy stretch for 30 seconds. Do not bounce.

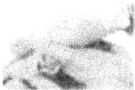

Knees to Chest Stretch for Lower Back (using a towel)

If it is difficult for you to reach your feet: Wrap a towel around the back of your knees and pull.

Lying Hamstring Stretch

Lie flat on your back and raise your left leg straight above you at 90 degrees, keeping your right leg flat on the floor. (If it is more comfortable or if you have lower back trouble, you can bend your right knee and put your right foot flat on the floor.) Hold your left leg with both hands right behind the knee for support. Pull slightly with your hands towards your head to feel a stretch along the back of your thigh. Hold for 30 seconds. Switch sides and repeat.

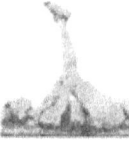

Lying Hamstring Stretch (using a towel)

If it is difficult for you to reach your knee without lifting your back off the ground, wrap a towel around the back of your knee and pull.

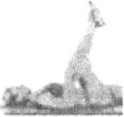

Outer Thigh Stretch for Iliotibial Band

Standing straight with hips, knees, and toes forward, raise your right foot off the floor. With your weight on your left leg, cross your right leg over your left foot, and stand with both feet flat on the floor. Lean through the left hip as you lean into your left leg, and bend at the waist over to the right side, with arms hanging at your sides. Push your right shoulder down to the floor, you should feel the stretch down the outside of your left thigh between your hip and knee bones. Hold for 30 seconds. Switch sides and repeat.

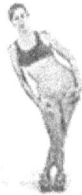

About the Author

DORRIS WOODS IS A LONG-TIME registered nurse. She holds a license in advanced clinical practice in nursing where she has taught and worked in nursing, hospital administration, and mental health. She is also a member of the National Association of Diabetes Educators.

She is the author of *Breaking Point: Fighting to End America's Teenage Suicide Epidemic!* She has written many articles on the topic and conducted workshops.

Dr. Woods earned her B.S. in Nursing and Psychology from Indiana University; a B.A. in Psychology from Regents College; two Master's Degrees in Nursing from UCLA - one in Pediatrics and Nursing Administration; the other in Mental Health. She also holds a Master's Degree in Counseling from California State University, Los Angeles; and a Ph.D. from Claremont Graduate University. She has done post-doctoral work at UCLA as well.

However, what she says she enjoys most is the ability to make a difference in the lives of people wherever she is and be able to comfortably relate to them. Write to her. She encourages your comments.

Dr. Woods is a widow and the mother of three children. She resides in Culver City, California with her loyal canine companion, Cookie.

Bibliography

Allen, Gloria. Personal communications on history of family diabetes, 2010.

Alley, Kirstie. "I've Let Myself Go," *People*, May 18, 2009: 51-57.

Blahnik, Jay. "Easy moves to rev the metabolism," *Los Angeles Times,* Feb. 26, 2007: F12.

Bollinger, Caroline. "Are You Sabotaging Your Diet?" *Prevention Magazine,* Nov. 2004: 138-140.

Brown, Eryn. "The surgeon general on healthy communities," *Health & Wellness,* March 13, 2011: A29.

Country Doctor Handbook, The. FC&A Medical Publishing (Peachtree, GA), 2010.

Deen, Darwin. "Metabolic Syndrome," The Family Doctor, June 15, 2004: 3 pp.

"Diabetes." *The Country Doctor Handbook,* FC&A Medical Publishing (Peachtree, GA), 2008: 90-107.

Diabetes Advisor 13, American Diabetes Association, 2006: 4 pp.

Fell, James S. "Interval training's fast track," *Los Angeles Times,* March 14, 2011: E6.

----------.   "To: Oprah; Re: Those guests," Los Angeles Times, Nov. 22, 2010: E6.

Graff, Cynthia, with Jerry Holderman. *Lean for Life "Daily Action Plan,"* Griffin Publishing Co. (Torrance, CA), 2001.

Greene, Bob. *Get with the Program,* Simon and Schuster (New York, NY), 2002.

Greider, Katharine. "The Real Fountain of Youth," *AARP Magazine,* Jan.-Feb. 2011: 10-14.

Grenfell, Monica. "Five days to a flatter stomach," *Family Circle*, Sept. 6, 2005: 82-83.

Grimmer, Brian. *Fitlinxx* (Shelton, CT), 2011.

Harrar, Sari. "Breakfast to beat diabetes," *Prevention Magazine,* March 2005: 39.

Harris Poll, *The Week*, August 3, 2007.

Maugh, Thomas H., II. "Diabetes study helps clear up contradictions on treatment*," Los Angeles Times*, June 9, 2008: A9-10.

Maugh, Thomas H., II. "Mr. Public Health Sparked Change," Los *Angeles Times*, April 12, 2012: A1.

"Metabolic Syndrome," *Family Doctor,* December 28, 2010: 1-2.

Pritikin, Nathan, and McGrady, Patrick M., Jr. *The Pritikin Program for Diet and Exercise,* Bantam Books (New York, NY), 1984. Roth,

Roth, Geneen. "Why Diets Don't Work," *Prevention Magazine,* March 2005: 89-91.

Shapiro, Howard M.   *Picture Perfect Weight Loss,* St. Martin's Press (New York, NY), 2000.

Teare, Tracy. "10 Ways to Walk Off Fat Faster," *Health.com*, November 2010: 97.

Thew, Jennifer. "Research Rounds: Obesity Costly to Society," available @ www.Nurse.com, June 4, 2007.

Torgovnick, Kate. "Lose the Weight for Good," *Good Housekeeping,*

March 2008: 151-155.

U.S. Department of Health and Human Services, Office of Women's Health. *The Healthy Woman: A Complete Guide for All Ages,* U.S. Government Printing Office (Washington, DC), 2010.

Williams, Brian. "Diabetes Has Reached Epidemic Proportions, Mainly Type Two," *NBC Evening News,* June 24, 2008.

Williams, Richard Allen. "What Black Women Need to Know About Heart Disease," *Los Angeles Sentinel,* Feb. 8, 2007: A-20.

www.ingramcontent.com/pod-product-compliance
Lightning Source LLC
Chambersburg PA
CBHW060235030426
42335CB00014B/1475